The Economics of Cancer Care

This book examines the interaction of economics and the delivery of cancer care in the global context. It analyses the causes of tension between those paying for care, those providing the care and those marketing drugs and devices for cancer. The concept and requirement for rationing is examined in different economic environments. As cancer increases in incidence and prevalence, the economics becomes a far more important subject than ever before. Written by a leading health economist and oncologist, this is the first comprehensive book on the economics of cancer and is a must have for health professionals and policy makers alike.

Nick Bosanquet is Professor of Health Policy at Imperial College London, UK, and is Special Advisor to the House of Commons Health Committee.

Karol Sikora is Visiting Professor of Cancer Medicine, Imperial College and Dean of the Brunel-Buckingham Medical School. He was formerly Chief of the WHO Cancer Programme.

We would like to thank Kate Bosanquet and Gill Miller for editorial assistance – much appreciated.

The Economics of Cancer Care

Nick Bosanquet

Professor of Health Policy
Imperial College

Karol Sikora

Dean, Brunel-Buckingham Medical School
Visiting Professor of Cancer Medicine, Imperial College

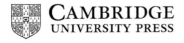
CAMBRIDGE
UNIVERSITY PRESS

CAMBRIDGE UNIVERSITY PRESS
Cambridge, New York, Melbourne, Madrid, Cape Town, Singapore, São Paulo

CAMBRIDGE UNIVERSITY PRESS
The Edinburgh Building, Cambridge CB2 2RU, UK

Published in the United States of America by Cambridge University Press, New York

www.cambridge.org
Information on this title: www.cambridge.org/9780521850070

© Cambridge University Press 2006

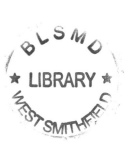

First published 2006

Printed in the United Kingdom at the University Press, Cambridge

A catalogue record for this publication is available from the British Library

Library of Congress Cataloguing in Publication data

ISBN-13   978-0-521-85007-0 hardback
ISBN-10   0-521-85007-X hardback

Cambridge University Press has no responsibility for the persistence or accuracy of
URLs for external or third-party internet websites referred to in this publication,
and does not guarantee that any content on such websites is, or will remain, accurate
or appropriate.

Every effort has been made in preparing this publication to provide accurate and up-to-date
information which is in accord with accepted standards and practice at the time of publication.
Although case histories are drawn from actual cases, every effort has been made to disguise the identities
of the individuals involved. Nevertheless, the authors, editors and publishers can make no warranties
that the information contained herein is totally free from error, not least because clinical standards are
constantly changing through research and regulation. The authors, editors and publishers therefore
disclaim all liability for direct or consequential damages resulting from the use of material contained in
this publication. Readers are strongly advised to pay careful attention to information provided by the
manufacturer of any drugs or equipment that they plan to use.

Contents

The challenge of cancer

Introduction

The title of this book, *The economics of cancer care*, raises important questions: Why are we interested in the economics of cancer care? And why are we especially interested *now*? This book will explore these two principal questions. First, it will review the current scientific literature on the economics of cancer care. The literature on the economics of cancer care is sparse and has received very little attention from the mainstream health economics field. Both the authors have reviewed the leading journals in the health economics and health policy field for the last 5 years. This has accrued 14,415 papers on the economics of cancer care since 1950, yet the subject remains noticeable by its absence in leading textbooks on cancer care. This compares with a total of over 16 million papers on cancer care and 85 million web sites on cancer. Only in a few specialised areas such as the cost-effectiveness of screening for breast cancer has there been much research.

Within health economics, most disease-specific work has been on the development of new drug therapies. The vast majority of the literature for the established programmes, especially in Europe, is generic and system-wide. The research has tended to focus on the cost-effectiveness of specific therapies with far less attention paid to the economics of choice at various stages of cancer treatment. However, there are fundamental reasons why the economic dimensions of cancer care need urgent attention.

Why the economics of cancer care deserve urgent attention

Increased prevalence due to longer survival is raising the cost of cancer care and creating new funding options for longer-term care and treatment programmes.

There is a continuous flow of new and very expensive therapies both in chemotherapy and in radiotherapy. The cost of drug therapies in oncology within the USA has risen by tenfold since 1991 compared to a rise of three-fold for all other therapies. Within radiotherapy a course of brachytherapy for prostate cancer can cost more than twice as much as the older therapy, which it replaced.

There are new and compelling reasons for re-engineering services; in order to improve communication with patients; provide longer-term care programmes; enable more targeted treatment; and invest in infrastructure and staff skills to effectively use the new direct therapies.

There are system-wide issues about how to achieve results from the developing model of care, which is at the core of a national cancer strategy. Specific initiatives to address the important problems associated with prevention and care over the past two decades can now be distilled into a single model, which all countries (north/south from Finland to Chile and east/west from Japan to the USA) are seeking to use. The main stages are:

- prevention,
- screening,
- treatment,
- continuing care and risk management,
- palliative care.

Most of the research has been conducted *within* stages yet increasingly there are important interactions *between* stages. Prevention is the most cost-effective way of reducing cancer: successful prevention will reduce the incidence of a type of cancer (smoking cessation has reduced the number of new cases of lung cancer). However, if prevention is not so easy (as in the case of prostate cancer, for example) then early detection from screening and the prospect of increasing survival rates create a plethora of problems to overcome.

Increasing screening is difficult and costly to organise on an effective basis. It requires a sizeable expansion in diagnostics and early-stage treatment. Treatment per patient is becoming increasingly costly as treatment combinations with different mixes of; surgery, radiotherapy and chemotherapy are being used. The area of treatment may begin to show greater differences within the "cancer industry", for example, between treatment for early-stage cancers detected through screening and the treatment of recurrent or faster acting types of cancer. These two "industries" may come to differ in their location, their staffing dynamics and their use of generics, as well as in their expected outcomes. The challenges of preventing recurrence, improving quality of life,

---

> **Box 1.1: The challenges for future cancer care**
>
> 1. Increasing the focus on prevention.
> 2. Improving screening and diagnosis.
> 3. New targeted treatments: How effective and affordable will they be?
> 4. Personalised medicine for cancer: delivering the diagnostics.
> 5. How people's expectations will translate into care delivery.
> 6. Reconfiguration of health services to deliver optimal care.
> 7. Geographical distribution of services: How close to people's homes?
> 8. Integrating public, private and charitable providers.
> 9. The impact of reconfiguration on professional territories.
> 10. The changes in the doctor–patient relationship.
> 11. Will society accept the potential financial burden?

and risk management, represent a rapidly growing area for cancer professionals where better communication with patients is urgently required. The model is likely to raise the need for long-term palliative care, which is currently under-provided in many existing systems of care (Box 1.1).

The prognosis for early-stage cancers has improved greatly over recent decades with the exception of lung cancer. Five-year survival rates for most early-stage cancers in the USA and Europe are now 90% or more (see Table 1.1). Further improvements are required both in survival and in improving the quality of life of survivors. However, these will require effective strategies to use the stage model to detect more cancers at an early stage and to target costly new therapies on "hard-to-cure" cancers. We write with optimism about the potential for further improvement and wherever possible we point to successes.

This book represents collaboration between an economist and a clinician. We have tried in the specific chapters to develop a dialogue between the "desire to cure every patient" spirit of the clinician, and the practical and more analytical questions raised by economists who recognise that there is not a "never-ending pot of money" to treat cancer, and that cancer is not the only cause of mortality and morbidity. Medical research and innovation develops the potential for new services: the take-up and speed of diffusion depends on economic incentives. Once an innovation is taken up the incentives may then contribute to the selection of different kinds of innovation. There are tensions between the absolutism of the medical demand for rapid take-up of costly new therapies and devices, and the counter forces of funding, regulation and provider

Table 1.1. US data on the benefits (5-year survival rates 1995–2000) of early diagnosis for major cancers

	All stages 5 year (%)	Localised 5 year (%)	Regional 5 year (%)	Distant 5 year (%)	Unstaged 5 year (%)
Prostate (M)	99.3	100.0	–	33.5	81.3
Colon and rectum*	63.4	90.5	67.9	9.4	35.2
Urinary bladder*	81.7	89.7	36.9	5.5	59.0
Non-Hodgkin lymphoma*	59.1	71.5	63.5	47.7	66.3
Breast (F)	87.7	97.5	79.1	20.4	56.7
Corpus and uterus (F)	84.4	95.8	67.0	22.5	56.0
Lung*	13.2	48.8	22.8	3.3	8.7
Cervix uteri (F)	72.7	92.2	55.1	17.2	59.2
Ovary (F)	44.0	94.2	77.6	28.5	23.9
Kidney and renal pelvis*	63.9	90.9	59.7	9.5	31.6
Stomach*	23.3	59.9	23.9	3.3	12.6

*Male and female combined.

Five-year survival rates, US

Type of cancer	Men			Women		
	1975–1979	1995–2000	Change (%)	1975–1979	1995–2000	Change (%)
All	42.7	64.0	21.3	56.6	64.3	7.7
Lung	11.6	13.6	2.0	16.6	17.2	0.6
Colon and rectum	50.3	63.7	13.4	52.3	63.1	10.8
Kidney and renal pelvis	51.8	63.7	12.1	51.3	63.9	12.6
Breast				74.9	87.7	12.8

Source: Jemal, 2004.[1]

resistance. For each treatment stage we have sought to identify both the opportunities in new therapies and the likely impact of economic incentives.

Our work with funders and professionals in Europe and the USA has convinced us that in order to improve services, change is inescapable. A new kind of cancer service is required and linear development of the old UK/European model will lead to great losses to patients and frustration to professionals as we fail to use new therapies effectively. New bottlenecks and communication problems will emerge as development of screening programmes, clinical governance and patient awareness raise demand faster than even enlarged services of the older types can deliver.

Our study draws on the work already being done to develop the new model. We pay tribute to the WHO's World Cancer Report which is our starting point. We hope to show that changing direction is both feasible and fundable. In the words of the Chinese sage Sun-Tzu:

> It is a matter of strategic positioning that the army that has this weight of victory on its side, in launching its men into battle, can be likened to the cascading of pent-up waters thundering through a steep gorge.[2]

The economic future of cancer care

Here we examine the economic future of cancer care; its incidence and prevalence; effects on global health; treatment methods; health and social care delivery structures; financial mechanisms; and its impact on society. We construct a series of alternative futures created by the potentially different levels of success of new technology, willingness to deal with the financial consequences and the capacity of society to adapt to the wider impact. We have tried to create a vision of the economic future of cancer and capture it in a concise format for health policy-makers, health and social care providers and purchasers, the health media, politicians and those professionals involved in delivering future cancer care.

Incidence of cancer set to increase

The incidence of cancer is increasing and is set to rise further. An ageing population will contribute more to this over the next two decades in Asia and Europe than in the USA. For the UK, incidence rates for all cancers will

Table 1.2. Mortality worldwide in 2000 – numbers of deaths (1000s)

Type of cancer	Male	Female	Both
Oesophagus	226.9	110.6	337.5
Colon/rectum	405.2	241.4	646.6
Liver	383.6	165.0	548.6
Pancreas	112.0	101.5	213.5
Lung	810.4	292.7	1031.1
Prostate	204.3	–	204.3
Breast	–	373.0	373.0
Cervix	–	233.4	233.4
Total	**3522.4**	**2686.3**	**6208.7**

Source: Parkin et al., 2001.[3]

rise by 2.5% per year in the over the age of 75 years. The age factor alone will increase patient numbers significantly over the next two decades. Improvements in screening and in diagnostics will also contribute to rising incidence especially for breast, prostate and colo-rectal cancers. Since 2000 it is estimated that 46% of men and 36% of women in the USA would be diagnosed with cancer in the course of their life spans. These probabilities are set to rise further with increasing incidence. Worldwide mortality is already high (Table 1.2).

Prevalence of cancer set to increase

Improved survival will increase prevalence especially as lung cancer (where survival rates are very poor) becomes less common. For the USA, the number of cancer survivors has risen from 3 million in 1970 to 10 million in 2000 and numbers are set to double as the full effects are felt of shifts to slower growing, less-aggressive cancers (prostate) and better survival through earlier detection. There will be a dramatic increase in global cancer prevalence over the next 20 years because of ageing populations.

Technological advances

The targeting of therapy will continue to improve and should achieve a more localised destruction of cancers with greater certainty and fewer adverse effects.

Minimally invasive surgery will reduce the need for routine organ resection without compromising survival. The application of sophisticated computer systems to radiotherapy planning will allow the precise shaping of beam delivery conforming exactly to the shape of the tumour. The increased precision of both these local modalities of tumour ablation will bring additional costs and the requirement for increasingly skilled technical manpower. Some of this time will come from new sources such as the outsourcing of complex radiotherapy planning through web-based links from the USA to groups of physicists and radiotherapists in India. The emergence of China as a massive information-based technocracy will have a huge impact on global service provision over the next decade simply because of its numbers of highly educated and skilled people working within a unique hierarchical social structure. Even so, costs of treatment are likely to increase both with rising incidence and increased intensity of treatment.

New chemotherapy drugs

Chemotherapy will be the area of greatest change. Expanding knowledge on the molecular genetics of cancer will impact on prevention, screening, diagnosis and treatment and drug discovery. There is much more understanding of the basic biological processes that become disturbed in cancer. We now know the key elements of growth factor binding, signal transduction, gene transcription control, cell cycle checkpoints, apoptosis and angiogenesis. This has widened options for drug discovery. The process is to identify novel targets known to be altered in cancer. This approach has already led to a record number of novel compounds currently in trials. Over the next decade there will be a marked shift in the types of agents used in the systemic treatment of cancer. Because we know the precise targets of these new agents, there will be a re-orientation in how we prescribe cancer therapy. Instead of defining drugs for use empirically and relatively ineffectively for different types of cancer, we will identify a series of molecular lesions in tumour biopsies. Future patients will receive drugs that target these lesions directly. The human genome project provides a vast repository of comparative information about normal and malignant cells. The new therapies will be more selective, less toxic and be given for prolonged periods of time, in some cases for the rest of the patient's life. We will convert cancer into a chronic, controllable illness similar to diabetes today.

Table 1.3. Summary of research on the value of medical technology changes

Condition	Years	Change in treatment costs	Outcome change	Value	Net benefit
Heart attack	1984–1998	$10,000	1 year increase in life expectancy	$70,000	$60,000
Low-birth weight infants	1950–1990	$40,000	12 year increase in life expectancy	$240,000	$200,000
Depression	1991–1996	$0 <$0	Higher remission probability at some cost for those already treated	More people treated with benefits exceeding costs	Highly positive
Cataracts	1969–1998	$0 <$0	Substantial improvements at no cost increase for those already treated	More people treated with benefits exceeding costs	Highly positive
Breast cancer	1985–1996	$20,000	4 months increase in life expectancy	$20,000	$0

Source: Cutler and McClellan, 2001.[4]

Individual cancer-risk assessment

Individual cancer-risk assessment will lead to tailored prevention messages and a specific screening programme to pick up early cancer. This will have far reaching implications for public health. Cancer preventive drugs will be developed to reduce the risk of further genetic deterioration. The use of gene arrays to monitor serum for fragments of DNA containing defined mutations could ultimately develop into an implanted gene chip. When a significant mutation is detected, the chip would signal the holder's home computer and set in train a series of investigations based on the most likely type and site of the primary tumour. Over the last two decades the evidence on the effectiveness of new therapies has been mixed. There have been some very positive gains for early-stage cancers but overall costs increased rapidly while survival showed only small increases. Thus Cutler and McClellan showed a contrast with other forms of therapy where results were highly favourable (Table 1.3).

New therapies are likely to face more stringent tests on value for money and cost-effectiveness.

Paying for cancer care

Cancer care was a declining proportion of total US health care costs from 1970 to 1995 but since then costs have started to rise rapidly.

The funding of cancer care will become a significant problem in all countries, rich and poor alike. Already we are seeing differences in access to the taxanes for breast and ovarian cancer, gemcitabine for lung and pancreatic cancer, and herceptin for breast cancer. Indeed, during the previous 2 years no less than five expensive therapies have been approved for marketing in the USA by the Food and Drug Administration. These drugs are only palliative, adding just a few months to life. The emerging compounds are likely to be far more successful, and their long-term administration will be considerably more expensive. Increased consumerism in medicine will lead to increasingly informed and assertive patients seeking out novel therapies and bypassing traditional referral pathways through global information networks. It is likely that integrated molecular solutions for cancer will develop, leading to far greater differences in access to treatment than at present. Novel financial structures constructed by consortia of the pharmaceutical, insurance and health care sectors will enable future patients to choose the levels of care they wish to pay for by insurance schemes or directly.

Projection of the future in cancer care

Eventually chemotherapy is likely to replace other treatment modalities for most cancers. Cancer will become a chronic, controllable illness rather like diabetes or hypertension today. Biomarkers of response will be used to guide, titrate and monitor chronic therapy. People living with cancer will receive care in an attractive hotel-like environment rather than a hospital, run by competing private sector providers. Global franchises will emerge using the web to disseminate treatment plans and control their quality. Many state health care systems will become regulators and insurers so eventually relinquishing their role as providers by 2010. This transition will bring new ethical and moral dilemmas. The alternative futures will be created by the interaction of four complex factors: technological success, society's willingness to pay, future health care delivery systems and the financial mechanisms that under-pin them.

Societal and political pressures

The ageing of the population will also mean that it is far more likely that individuals affected by cancer and their carers' will have multiple diseases. This will affect both the treatment opportunities and the care services needed during and after treatment. Predictions for the main causes of death and disability 20 years hence suggest that worldwide, the top five causes of death will be; ischaemic heart disease, cerebrovascular disease, chronic obstructive pulmonary disease, respiratory infections and lung cancer. Disability will be mainly due to cerebrovascular disease, ischaemic heart disease, cancers and neuropsychiatric conditions. It is debatable whether lengthening life expectancy will be disability-free, or whether the added years of life will bring with them more years of life lived with disability. If the latter, demand for tending care will escalate as age-related conditions including cancer evolve from acute to chronic.

The rise in age-related disease and demand for holistic care of the individual will be accompanied by an age-related decline in the workforce: current proposals to abandon a statutory retirement age will not stop us all getting older. The health workforce in developed countries will shrink as cohorts of nurses and general practitioners (GPs) become eligible for retirement. The growth of single-person households will reduce the amount of family care available. The workforce available for the "tending trades" will continue to diminish, unless perhaps offset by migration from the new member states of the European union (EU) with youthful populations, the domestication of health technologies, shifting of professional role boundaries and employment of those above current retirement age.

Wealth and cancer incidence

The world is in a period of health transition. Communicable disease (infections) as a major cause of suffering and death is giving way to new epidemics of non-communicable disorders such as cardiovascular disease, diabetes and cancer. Different countries are in different stages of this transition depending on their age structure and economy. Some countries are faced with a double burden with increasing infection problems compounded by surging cancer rates. This is fuelled in part by the globalisation of unhealthy lifestyles. The pace of this change is difficult to predict. The world population is ageing with a predicted average longevity of 73 years by the year 2020 compared with 66 in 1997. It has been estimated that there will be a greater than 100% increase in the population aged over 65 in more than 30 countries. Ageing alone will dramatically increase the cancer burden.

The next 25 years will be a time of unprecedented change in the way in which we will control cancer. However, the optimal organisation of prevention, detection and care programmes, as well as treatment services, is a universal problem in all economic environments. There are clear relationships between current cancer incidence figures for different countries with their relative wealth. Using demographic data we can also predict changes in cancer incidence over the next 25 years and relate this change to relative wealth.

Longevity and wealth

Figure 1.1 examines the relationship between life expectancy at birth for both men and women, and wealth of the 155 countries studied. There is a clear relationship between increasing gross national product (GNP) and longer life. There are relatively large gains for small increases in per capita GNP in dollars (pcGNP$) in the poorer countries, reflecting reduced infant and childhood mortality. Above a pcGNP$ of 1000 the proportional gain in longevity is markedly reduced. This almost certainly reflects the importance of basic measures such as vaccination, good water supply, improved health education and access to simple medical care. After this longevity continues to increase with wealth but increasingly slowly reflecting the biological determinants that cause disease and death in all human populations.

There are two interesting clusters (Figure 1.1). The first are those countries where longevity is significantly less than expected for their relative wealth with a pcGNP$ of above 2000 but a longevity of less than 60 years. These are three African countries: Namibia, Botswana and Gabon. The high level of HIV-related disease is the factor responsible for this. The second cluster are those states with a higher than expected longevity of greater than 65 years but a pcGNP$ of below 1000. These include: Egypt, Thailand, Honduras,

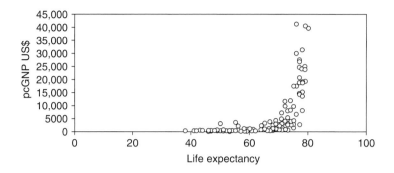

Figure 1.1   Longevity and wealth.

Nicaragua, Vietnam, Mongolia, Indonesia, China, Surinam, Kyrgistan, Sri Lanka, Tajikstan, Turkmenistan, Uzbekistan, Armenia, Georgia, Azerbaijan, Albania, Macedonia and the Solomon Islands. Common factors are efficient public health systems, low infant and childhood mortality and an integrated primary care system. A further confounding factor are the relatively recent reductions in pcGNP$ in these countries caused by changes in external factors and the political structures in such countries. Clearly there is a long incubation period between the factors responsible for longevity and the outcome. Major changes over the last decade will have considerable impact over the next 25 years.

Figures 1.2 and 1.3 show the relationship between wealth and cancer in men and women. There is a clear correlation between increasing wealth and cancer incidence. This is almost certainly due to the influence of tobacco and dietary factors as well as other more complex lifestyle factors together with increased longevity of the population. Exceptions include a cluster with a pcGNP$ of greater than 5000 and a cancer incidence of less than 150 per

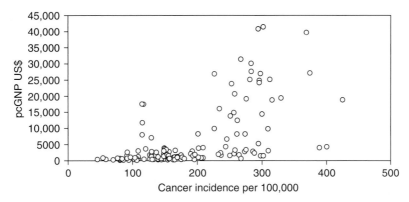

Figure 1.2   Cancer incidence in men.

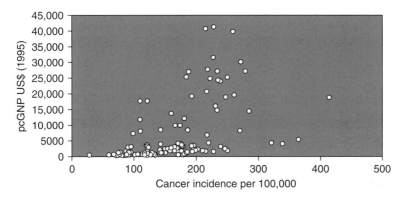

Figure 1.3   Cancer incidence in women.

100,000. These are all Arabian Gulf states. This almost certainly reflects the benefit of the traditional lifestyle maintained by the majority of the population. The second cluster are the former socialist countries of Europe, certain former Soviet republics and South Africa where the cancer incidence exceeds 250 per 100,000 but the pcGNP$ is less than 5000. This reflects increased longevity due to good public health and efficient health care systems, a Western lifestyle and again a reduction in real pcGNP$ due to political factors. Figures 1.4 and 1.5 show the ratios of cancer incidence in 2020:1990 for both men and women correlated to relative wealth. The largest changes in incidence are clearly predicted for poorer countries with a good correlation

Table 1.4. Incidence of cancer – all sites by world area 2000

	ASR (World) per 100,000 pop male	ASR (World) per 100,000 pop female	Cumulative risk (age 0–64) male	Cumulative risk (age 0–64) female
More developed countries	301.0	218.3	14.4	12.5
Less developed countries	153.8	127.4	8.2	8.0
World	201.9	157.8	10.0	4.2

Source: Parkin et al., 2001.

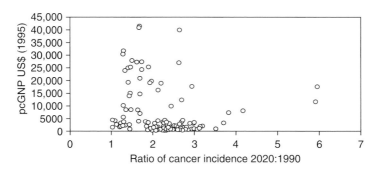

Figure 1.4   Change in cancer incidence in men by 2020.

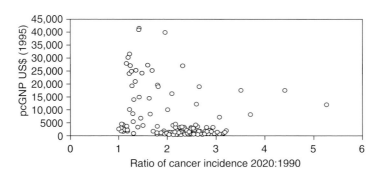

Figure 1.5   Change in cancer incidence in women by 2020.

between poverty and greatly increased incidence. Countries with the greatest increase will have the least facilities to deal with the health care problems posed by the disease.

Cancer is currently a disease of wealthy nations: (Table 1.4) but over the next 25 years there will be major changes. A much greater increase in cancer is predicted for poorer countries that lack adequate resources currently to treat the disease. Furthermore, likely technological advances will bring greater treatment success but in many cases at a price beyond that affordable by state-driven medical services in many countries. We could potentially prevent a quarter of all cancers simply by applying existing knowledge. A third are curable using today's technology and this can be confidently predicted to rise by one-half over the next 25 years. The appropriate expertise has to be in the right place at the right time and widely accessible. For those that cannot be cured, effective palliation of symptoms, especially pain, should be a basic human right. We need to take effective action now to reduce cancer incidence as much as possible. For many countries this will be the only economically realistic route. An effective strategy accompanied by political will, skilled persuasion, good media relations as well as international professional and industrial collaboration will be vital to achieve this.

Aims of this book

The critical question that we ask is: Can the goal of achieving excellence in cancer services only be attainable for the minority of affected patients and within a privileged few nations? Here, we make the case for optimism about the opportunities for improving use of scarce resources across cancer prevention and care. Reliable and effective services are becoming more feasible and fundable in smaller centres as well as capital cities and in middle-income countries. Opportunities for outstanding achievement are no longer limited to a few major cancer centres. The professional and human commitment of staff in cancer care can be used more effectively to improve processes and outcomes for most patients in many countries. Cancer services could surprise the world by a decade of improving outcomes, process and patient confidence. We can estimate the progress already made over the last two decades, but much more needs to be done.

Mortality from cancer now counts for a high proportion of premature (under 70-year olds) deaths from 25% to 30% overall for all and 40% plus for women. These proportions are likely to increase further as coronary heart disease reduces, and with increasing incidence of breast and sometimes lung cancer. Improved cancer care would be a significant investment programme. For most developed countries, cancer is one of the three most important causes of years lost from the workforce. With economic concerns about workforce reductions as population's age, this becomes an economic as well as a humanitarian issue. Patients who have suffered cancer and recovered are often in poor health and a recent national survey sponsored by the National Cancer Institute showed that "Compared with matched control subjects, cancer survivors had poorer outcomes across all burden measures."[5] There are new concerns about queuing and rationing of care, which are beginning to emerge in insurance-funded as well as tax-funded systems. There are new challenges in building partnerships with patients who express higher levels of concern about lack of information. Cancer services have often scored unusually low in survey evidence on quality of communication with patients.

In the future, increased prevalence, which is expected to rise 50% or more over the next decade, will put further pressure on process and outcomes. Even if there are some increases in real funding on health services such numbers point to a situation in which real expenditure per patient will rise little, and where funding is particularly tight, real funding per patient will actually decline. Even where funding seems to be available there will be a scarcity of qualified and experienced staff. There may be funding but little to buy with it. We have argued that every Minister of Health should have a notice on his wall: "I cannot increase the number of experienced staff in my term of office", and this applies to cancer laboratories where high levels of knowledge are required for risk assessment and treatment planning. Sustained improvement in system performance is essential. We aim to contribute to it through our review of the economic evidence, which is now extensive and international but dispersed.

We develop three key themes:

1. A new model is beginning to emerge for cancer care, which seeks to explore the linkages between main stages rather than a series of unconnected initiatives in screening or radiotherapy. The full cancer programme now covers prevention, screening, surgery, radiotherapy, chemotherapy, follow-up care and palliative care.

We seek evidence both on the economics of each stage but also on the impacts that change in any one stage has on others. We also explore the opportunities for using integration to raise "productivity" in the system.

2. Cancer services should make full use of new economic incentives. The work of Herzlinger and more recently of the Organisation for Economic Cooperation and Development (OECD) has explored and documented the powerful gains for better care that can be achieved by using economic incentives and competition. Such change can open up access to IT technology and expertise from the global economy. The tendency in difficult areas of care such as cancer services has however been to shy away from these new incentives and to recoil back towards a public sector national monopoly. We challenge this reaction particularly in view of the strong evidence that the outstanding outcomes achieved and recognised across the USA are partly related to greater competition between providers, which has contained cost and improved access.

3. There are new opportunities for international collaboration and learning. The extension of clinical trials to many more countries has been a most practical and positive way of improving services and prepares the way for an extension of international audit and comparison. One message is likely to be that some systems have been able to achieve strikingly good results with very limited resources. The recent Eurocare 3 Survey has shown that for patients diagnosed in 1990–1994, outcomes were being achieved in the Czech Republic, Slovakia and Poland that were two-thirds as good as those achieved in the USA with a small fraction of the resources.[6] In South America, Chile has given an outstanding example of how to develop a national cancer strategy.

The WHO's World Cancer Report broke new ground in showing both the diversity of the challenges faced and their predicted expansion in the near future. There are now opportunities to develop specific targeted strategies for problems such as cervical cancer in the Andean Republics of Latin America and lung cancer in Central Europe. International leadership in cancer care used to be concentrated in a few countries and a few centres: now as in so many other areas of activity there is greater communication with the chance for unexpected new therapies and improvements to emerge from new clusters.

REFERENCES

1. Jemal A. et al. (2004) Report to the nation on the status of cancer 1975–2001, with a special feature regarding survival. *Cancer* 101: 3–27.
2. Sun-Tzu. (1993) *The Art of Warfare*. Ballantine Books, NY.
3. Parkin D., Bicat F. and Devida S. (2001) Cancer burden in the year 2000. The global picture. *European Journal of Cancer* 37: 4–66.
4. Cutler D. and McClellan M. (2001) Is technological change worth it? *Health Affairs* 20: 11–29.
5. Yabroff K.R. et al. (2004) Burden of illness in cancer survivors: Findings from a population based national sample. *Journal of the National Cancer Institute* 96(17): 1322–1330.
6. Sant M. et al. (2000) Eurocare-3: Survival of cancer patients diagnosed 1990–94, results and commentary. *Annals of Oncology* 14(suppl 5): 61–118.

2

Prevention

Introduction

When assessing cost effectiveness, health economics often has to report on the high costs of activities presenting barriers to wider adoption. More rarely, problems loom on the demand side with a low take up of a programme, which costs little to organize. In the case of prevention, it is not the cost of the programmes that have been the main issue but rather achieving results. Prevention of cancer is immensely attractive as a goal but so far has led to more modest results than were predicted or indeed have been achieved in preventing coronary heart disease (CHD).

There have certainly been some gains within current prevention programmes principally in tobacco control. These include reductions in lung cancer coming about quite rapidly among middle-aged males in the US, UK, and more recently in Poland. Without such measures, total incidence and mortality might have shown a continuing increase rather than stabilising. International comparisons suggest that active tobacco control policies can reduce cancer mortality for men some 20% below the levels found within a nation of persistent smokers. Reducing smoking is the most effective and immediate way of reducing mortality from cancer. Yet lung cancer still results in over 50% of premature life years lost worldwide because of poor survival rates amongst those suffering the disease. Considering that prevention has a surprisingly rapid impact on reducing the toll, the dividend from successful prevention policies could be large. If there is to be a realistic chance of reducing mortality by 20% worldwide over the next decade then prevention policies are going to have to play a large part in cancer care. There is no other realistic way to achieve significant reductions in mortality so quickly.

The aims of this chapter are to:

- present international evidence on the economics of prevention in the first policy wave;
- set out some possible directions for a further policy wave that might produce stronger results in the specific area of cancer prevention.

There are very strong arguments for prevention programmes in preventing other diseases especially CHD and diabetes and in promoting well being, but we need to question whether different targeting of policies could achieve better results in the specific area of cancer. Certainly, the US National Cancer Institute's (NCI) broad goals of reducing mortality will be hardly attainable without a very distinct improvement in the productivity of prevention.

The economics of prevention: the balance sheet so far

The main policy directions for the last decade have been towards comprehensive tobacco control programmes. In other areas such as diet and exercise programmes, attempts have been tentative and inspirational, but in relation to smoking there is experience with specific and wide ranging initiatives that have been successfully implemented. Tobacco control programmes were first developed in Scandinavia and later in the US. After the initial warnings given in the Surgeon General's Report of 1964 there were some moves including banning of advertising. The main emphasis was on providing information about the effects of smoking in causing serious illness.

From 1977 onwards, the emphasis shifted and the Federal Government and Congress set a more ambitious target, raised important new issues and promoted a wider range of policy initiatives. First Health Education and Welfare Secretary Califano, and then Surgeon General Everett Koop, developed a much greater sense of urgency and a greater willingness to tackle interests.

New targets

In 1978 the Secretary of Health, Education and Welfare announced a major government initiative against smoking. Smoking was called the "Public Health Enemy Number One." By 1980, "the Department of Public Health had refined this into a definite objective of reducing smoking to below 25%

among adults by 1990." By 1984 the Surgeon General had set an even more ambitious target of a smoke-free society by the year 2000.

The Surgeon General broadened the analysis of the consequences on health of smoking well beyond the original issue of lung cancer. A Report in 1983 dealt exclusively with smoking and cardio-vascular disease, and a Report in 1984 analysed the relationship between smoking and obstructive lung disease, but the most important new issue was that of passive smoking. The 1986 Report broke new ground in dealing with the health consequences of involuntary smoking. The issue led to an important change of emphasis. Smokers were not just damaging their own health but that of other people as well. By the late 1980s the Surgeon General had been able to document: "the central role of cigarette smoking as a massive, preventable personal, and public health problem[1]". As well as accounting for 30% of all cancers, smoking was a "major" cause of cardio-vascular disease, aortic aneurysms, bronchitis, chronic obstructive pulmonary disease (COPD), and poor development in pregnancy.

New initiatives

The anti-smoking campaigns in the 1960s and 1970s had focused on information concerned with the consequences of smoking on health. The 1980s saw the use of price and tax policy. In 1982, Congress temporarily doubled the Federal Excise Tax on cigarettes to 16 cents per pack to be effective from 1983–1985. The increase was later extended permanently.

In 1988, California voters passed a referendum raising the cigarette excise tax to 25 cents per pack. Revenues were set aside for public health use. The principal manoeuvre in the 1980s was to raise the price of cigarettes. The first wave of price changes had very positive results. From November 1st 1981 to November 1st 1984 the average retail price of cigarettes rose from 70 to 98 cents, a real terms increase above the general rate of inflation of 26%. "Based on an overall price elasticity of 0.47 for adults and teenagers, per capita consumption should have declined by about 12% over the period. Department of Agriculture data show a decline of 11–12%. Although per capita consumption had been slowly declining at the rate of about 1% per annum since the mid-1970s, the very rapid acceleration in the rate of decline following the excise tax increases and associated price increases served as

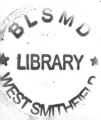

further evidence that excise taxes may be a potent tool to discourage smoking.[1]" However, this policy instrument has become much less effective. Cross border trade in cigarettes has made it very difficult to secure continuing cigarette price increases in real terms. Canada and Scandinavia have found that importation of cheaper cigarettes from the US and the Baltic Republics respectively has undermined attempts to raise prices. Even where there have been further real-term price increases the results have been disappointing. One recent study of California showed results very different from the 1980s when price increases led to a decline in prevalence from 26.3% to 21.2% in the period 1987–1990. Price increases in 1998 and 1999 produced no change in prevalence although they did bring about some fall in consumption per smoker. The study concluded: "Since smoking prevalence is significantly lower than it was a decade ago, price increases are becoming less effective as an inducement for hard core smokers to quit, although they may respond by decreasing consumption.[2]" The American Cancer Society has recently defined the goals of comprehensive tobacco control:

- prevent the initiation of tobacco use among young people;
- promote quitting among young people and adults;
- eliminate non-smokers exposure to environmental tobacco smoke;
- identify and eliminate the disparities in tobacco use and its effects on different population groups.

Table 2.1 displays recent levels of smoking in the US for 2001.

These figures give a balance sheet of results of the first phase of prevention and the optimism created by the Surgeon General's 1989 Report "Reducing the Health Consequence of Smoking. 25 Years of Progress" has faded considerably. The figures illustrate three important points.

The target of reducing smoking prevalence to 25% was reached, but 10 years late. By 2000, the US was still a long way from reaching the aim of a smoke free America. The great hopes of the Koop era are sadly very far from being realised.

Smoking rates are still high in the age groups where increasing age increases risk, from 25 to 44 and 45 to 64. Smoking prevalence would look even less impressive if the focus was just on the prime adult group excluding the retired population where smoking rates are 10% or less. Smokers with higher education have given up but smoking rates are as high as 40% among

Table 2.1. Current cigarette use amongst adults aged 18 years and above, US, 2001

Age group (years)	% of men	% of women	% of total population
18–24	30.4	23.4	26.9
25–44	27.3	24.5	25.8
45–64	26.4	21.4	23.8
65 or above	11.5	9.2	10.1
Number of years of education			
8 or fewer	24.2	13.4	18.6
9–11	39.5	29.8	34.3
12	29.3	23.4	26.1
13–15	26.6	22.1	24.2
16 or more	13.3	11.2	12.3
More than 16	9.0	10.0	9.5
Total	25.2	20.7	22.8

Source: American Cancer Society.

groups with less education where people are more likely to have multiple risk factors. For people with less education smoking prevalence was slightly higher in the US in 2001 than it had been in 1987 (35.7% in 1987 and 39.5% in 2001).

However, there have been some real successes. From 1965 to 2001, consumption of cigarettes per capita fell from 4345 to 2047 representing very substantial reduction in risk. Smoking rates in the two States with most intensive programmes held out some hope of further decline (16.4% in California in 2001 and 19.0% in Massachusetts) but in general the result were disappointing. Even in the promised land of Massachusetts 27.7% of people with low education were smokers.

International evidence also shows how difficult it has been to reduce smoking enough to achieve the results necessary to reduce mortality. Comparing countries with weak or ineffective policies on tobacco control such as Germany and Denmark with countries such as Sweden and the UK demonstrates that there have even some reductions in cancer mortality, averaging around 10% (Table 2.2). For example, German mortality from cancer for

Table 2.2. Comparison between different countries' smoking rates and death rates from lung cancer

Country	Smoking rate among all adults (%)	Mortality rate from lung cancer per 100,000 of the population 1999–2000	
		Men	Women
USA	25.7	161.8	116.4
UK	26.0	171.0	128.0
Germany	34.0	176.6	116.9
Sweden	22.0	137.9	104.0
Denmark	38.0	184.9	144.0
Australia	21.0	150.9	103.2

Source: American Cancer Society.

men was 9% higher than in the US for 2001. Across the whole range of countries, mortality from lung cancer was 26.5% lower in Sweden than in Denmark, which showed that it was possible to make very significant gains.

Of course there are many other variables which affect cancer incidence apart from the presence or absence of tobacco control policies, but the international data do at least show a continued high level of mortality even in countries where there have been considerable efforts to reduce smoking. At the very least, such findings should surely intensify the search for more effective measures to reduce smoking.

Tobacco control in the UK

Smoking prevalence among males in the UK started from an even higher level than in the US – at 60% in the early 1960s compared with 50% in the US. During the 1970s and 1980s there was a rapid fall in smoking prevalence in both countries. However, for the UK the decline in prevalence did not continue in the 1990s, not even at a slower rate. More recently there has been a slight decline to 25%. Average prevalence rates have tended to be higher for manual workers (32%) compared to those in non-manual occupations (21%). Among women, smoking rates have doubled over the last two decades and at 25% are now just below those for men, which are 28%. Similarly to the US, the amount of further reduction since the late 1980s must be considered disappointing. At the current rate of progress it will be difficult to achieve even the modest target of reducing smoking prevalence to 24% by 2004 and even more difficult to achieve the target of reducing smoking prevalence among manual groups to 26% in 2010. More ambitious targets were recommended as part of the Wanless fully engaged scenario.[3]

"In 2001, 27% of adults smoked according to the General Household Survey. The Government set a target of 24% smoking prevalence for 2010 in *Smoking Kills* based on the General Household Survey data, but the full-engaged scenario assumed that in that time scale, Californian levels of smoking (17%) would be met. If it is then assumed that the downward trend continued at half that rate in the years to 2022, smoking prevalence then would be 11%. That would represent a decrease of more than one half in smoking prevalence in 20 years, of about 6.2 million fewer smokers."

On the other hand, on current trends, if the reduction in smoking prevalence experienced in the adult population between 1993 and 2001 were continued until 2022, prevalence would remain marginally above 20%. The quantification of smoking reduction for the fully engaged model shows the scale of the challenge and illustrates the point that attainment of previously set targets would not be enough.

Tobacco control in Europe

With the exception of the UK and Scandinavia, the profile of change in Europe compared to the US has been rather different. There was little fall in smoking in the 1970s and 1980s even among the middle classes. Across the European Union (EU) in 1988, rates of smoking among doctors were comparable with those among EU citizens generally (36%).[4] In Spain (44%) and Italy (41%) smoking was more common among doctors than in the population generally. Since then there has been a slight fall in smoking rates by higher income groups and older males, but rising smoking rates among younger women has offset this so total prevalence has remained unchanged at around 35%.[5] In Scandinavia, there has been little progress particularly in Denmark where, in spite of high prices and strong anti-tobacco programmes, smoking rates remain some of the highest in the developed world.

There have, however, been some positive policy changes. In 2000, the signing of the World Health Organisation (WHO) Framework Convention set out comprehensive measures covering excise taxes, labelling, and the banning of smoking in both work and public places. This contributed to greater policy activity, particularly in France and Ireland. In France, the main development was a rise in excise taxes, which doubled the price of cigarettes over a 3-year period. Ireland led the way in terms of active bans on smoking in public places. Political decisions emerged at a time when personal decision-making (voluntarily giving up) seemed to be having little impact on reducing smoking prevalence. By 2004, smoking prevalence across Europe was at the same level as in the US 30 years earlier.

The economics of prevention: future

In 1989, the Surgeon General's Report entitled *25 Years of Progress* set out a framework to reduce the health consequences of smoking. We now seem a long way from the extraordinary achievement of the Koop era when it could be hoped that, "the ashtray is following the spittoon into oblivion". The stalling of progress in reducing smoking rates has a particularly negative impact on cancer prevention, as changes in other variables – diet, lifestyle, and air pollution may have led to continued and more immediate progress in cardio-vascular and respiratory disease.

The current moves to comprehensive anti-tobacco control policies certainly need to be maintained and strengthened. Without them, rising real incomes and changes in consumer tastes might have led to significant increases in smoking prevalence. But new actions are needed for the long and short term to give more impetus to the aim of reducing smoking. For the longer term, a ban on smoking in public places is essential if there is to be any chance of reducing prevalence over the next 5 years. On international evidence this might lower smoking prevalence 4–5 percentage points and it would have a positive effect in raising the prominence of the whole issue.

Such a change in prevalence would however affect cancer risk only over the longer term. New initiatives are needed to bring about more immediate results. As the recent Report from HEW on *Women, Tobacco and Cancer: An Agenda for the 21st century* set a relevant objective: "Overall goal: Develop new and more effective interventions to prevent and treat tobacco use and

environment tobacco smoke (ETS) exposure among women and girls, especially in populations at greatest risk."[6] As long ago as 1978 the NCI began a
major shift in funding priorities towards behavioural patterns and there is
now much evidence on the gains to smoking cessation programmes.

The key challenge is to develop stronger personal motivation to reduce
risk. At present, risk factors as defined by epidemiologists seem to be out of
line with risk factors as seen by individuals. For epidemiologists smoking
presents as a massive risk factor for cancer, yet most individuals seem to take
little notice. One challenge is to get across a clearer definition of high risk.
Concern about initiation by younger smokers has reduced the funding and
energies available for cessation programmes among older smokers. Yet for
cancer the risk faced by smokers are low until age 50+. Quitting smoking in
the 40–45 age group can make a very big difference to cancer risk. For smokers in their 50s the risk is very large and personal – nearly one in two are
going to die prematurely of smoking related disease.

Marketing smoking cessation

We present here the economics of a targeted and sustained effort to reach
smokers in the 40–45 age group around such themes as: "Do you want to see
your grand children?" For the UK, this would involve targeting a group of
approximately 2 m people in the 40–45 age range. Within this group some
500,000 are likely to be smokers. Thus there would be about 20 smokers on
each GP list.[7] Some of these would already be included in programme for
reducing risk of CHD and Diabetes but without allowing for any cost offsets
it would be possible to organise a fairly intensive and personal programme
for £100 a head. For the whole age group the costs nationally would be £50 m.
If around 10% of smokers were to give up over and above the expected
decline in prevalence this would produce a saving of 250,000 life years at
cost of £200 per life year. Even if only one extra smoker gave up per practice
this would produce a cost per life year of £400. Raising motivation among
high-risk groups is vital to achieve successful results over the next decade.

The evidence base is now much more secure for the development of this
personal targeted process. At the time of the Surgeon General's Report there
was on-going research about models of commitment and release from
smoking. Now there is strong and widely accepted evidence that smoking is

---

Box 2.1: Cancer prevention
1. Health inequity exists in smoking related diseases.
2. Complex genetic – environment interactions will be identified.
3. Novel prevention strategies are likely to lead to similar inequity.
4. Creating meaningful incentives to reduce risk will be essential.
5. Tailored messages will have greater power to change lifestyles.
6. Anti-inflammatory drugs could be effective cancer preventives.
7. Biomarkers of risk will enhance the validation of preventive drugs and compliance in the use of these drugs.
8. Novel providers of risk assessment and correction will emerge.
9. Public education is the key to cancer prevention.
10. Risk banding of populations will lead to specific tailored programmes.

---

addictive. Reducing disease burden is one of the most challenging aspects in the overall economics of cancer. What we do today about prevention will have a major impact on how many cancers there will be as well as their types in future. In England alone there are 225,000 new cases of cancer each year with 120,000 people dying from it. Compare that with the 3000 deaths in road traffic accidents just to get the scale. Probably between two-thirds and three-quarters of all cancers are preventable. In theory, we could prevent 80,000 of the 120,000 people dying of cancer just by using current knowledge. Half of these preventable deaths will be smoking related. Smoking, of course, causes many other diseases of the heart, lungs and arteries. The total number of people dying from smoking in the UK exceeds 120,000. A long-term smoker has a 50% chance of dying from a smoking induced illness and a 25% chance of dying under the age of 70. If there is to be a serious chance of reducing mortality from cancer by 15–20% over the next 10 years then reductions in smoking rates are essential. There is no other route that can deliver reductions in mortality as quickly or with such low expenditure of resources (Box 2.1).

Poland developed strong policies for reducing smoking in the mid-1990s, and already by the year 2000, lung cancer mortality among men had fallen 15% and mortality was 30% lower than in Hungary. The reduction in lung cancer rates for Poland can be estimated to produce a gain of 40,000 lives saved in the 35–69 age groups over the next decade. Similar gains have been made by states within the US. California and Massachusetts now have smoking rates that are 50% lower than those in Kentucky and there has been a striking change in relative mortality from lung cancer.

Diet and cancer

The tightest evidence on cancer causation is with smoking because it is easy to quantify. A smoker knows exactly when they started. They know how many they smoked a day and when they gave up. The connection between diet and cancer is a lot more complicated. Even remembering what people had the previous day can be quite difficult but there is sound evidence for a relationship between diet and cancer. Obesity is now linked with colon, post-menopausal breast, endometrial and with kidney cancer. Others will almost certainly be added to that list. The evidence linking increased cancer incidence to physical inactivity is also growing. An estimated 3 million people get cancer because of diet – breast cancer, colo-rectal cancer, hepatoma and several others. The difficulty with the dietary relationship is its complexity. It is not just what we eat but also what we do not eat, how the food is prepared and how it relates to hormonal status that matters – a very complex set of factors. A fascinating study investigating this issue is the European Prospective Investigation of Cancer (EPIC) conducted by the WHO. It will be published in about 3 years time. It uses Europe as a natural laboratory with a gradient of diets – the high fat-eating people in Scandinavia in the north to the olive oil culture of the Mediterranean in Southern Italy. It is prospectively collecting data from over half a million people and correlating cancer incidence to dietary history. The results will have profound social and political significance at a time of major turmoil in the food industry.

For diet and prevention there has been little success in identifying patterns of causation that would affect all or most cancers. The recent 10-year follow-up of the US nurses and health professionals panels showed that there was a strong relationship between fruit and vegetable intake and cardiovascular disease but no relationship between diet and cancer.[8] More success has seemed likely in research on some specific types of cancer. There would seem to be a strong association from the international evidence between per capita consumption of meat and colo-rectal cancer mortality. However, "mortality rates for colo-rectal cancer are similar in western vegetarians and comparable non-vegetarians.[9]" As with the impact of high fibre diets on colo-rectal cancer, the associations between meat eating and cancer have seemed less clear as research has progressed. However, possible links between consumption of dairy products and breast cancer now provide an important new area for research. The clearest and most sustained association is between obesity and cancer. A recent review concludes:

Since the 1981 Doll and Peto review on diet and cancer mortality, about one third of cancers have generally been thought to be related to dietary factors. More recent evidence suggests that this number may be too high, but a revised quantitative estimate is beyond the scope of this review. Among the diet-related factors, overweight/obesity convincingly increases the risks of several common cancers. After tobacco, overweight/obesity appears to be the most important avoidable cause of cancer in populations with Western patterns of cancer incidence. Among non-smoking individuals in these populations, avoidance of overweight is the most important strategy for cancer prevention.[9]

Given the increase in obesity for many nations including most of Europe and the US, the main challenge in prevention will be to prevent a significant increase in cancer as a result of dietary factors.

Cancer and infections

1.5 million people globally a year develop cancers due to infection. Papillomavirus, Epstein–Barr virus and hepatitis B virus all cause cancer and although immunisation strategies are possible with today's technology, in practice it is difficult to pull the resources together for economic and political reasons. In the Gambia for example a randomised trial funded by the WHO showed that hepatitis B immunisation costing less than $2 per child would drastically lower the subsequent incidence of hepatoma. In Banjul, the capital of the Gambia, the most prevalent form of cancer is hepatoma and it is universally lethal. There is simply no effective treatment anywhere in the world. But politicians simply cannot afford to have long-term aims because of electoral cycles so spending $2 makes no sense to them for a benefit in 40 years time.

Tailored chemoprevention and its economic consequences

We are at the threshold of developing the potential for effective cancer chemoprevention and the pharmaceutical industry is beginning to awaken to this new opportunity. There are specific chemopreventives such as tamoxifen for breast cancer and finasteride for prostate cancer. It is now clear that the development of many cancers is associated with inflammation. Inflammation switches on the cyclo-oxygenase II (Cox 2) enzyme and there are several inhibitors available that are already licenced for clinical use as anti-inflammatory analgesics. Aspirin, many non-steroidal anti-inflammatory drugs (NSAIDs), as well more specific Cox 2 inhibitors, similar to NSAIDs but without the gastric irritant side effects, are in routine clinical use for chronic inflammatory conditions such as arthritis. The inflammatory process switches off the local immune response so reducing immune surveillance for disordered cells and switches on growth factors leading to angiogenesis, a process crucial to cancer formation.

The role of inflammation in cancer causation is ubiquitous. Lung cancers occur in people who have had longstanding chronic bronchitis. Oesophageal and stomach cancers are associated with chronic helicobacter pylori infection. This can be eradicated by antibiotics. Chronic inflammation due to hepatitis B or C leads to hepatoma. It takes decades to lead to increased cancer risk but could be an interesting point for intervention. There have been many prospective trials followed by meta-analyses showing that aspirin above a dose of 300 mg a day will reduce the risk of colon cancer by about 50%. Indeed most solid cancers show a reduction of around 20%. The use of less toxic, more potent anti-inflammatory agents in high-risk individuals could have a potentially enormous potential to impact on cancer incidence.

The comparison to the development of cholesterol lowering agents – the statins – is interesting. There are two major differences: firstly, a well-documented biomarker (serum cholesterol) also acts as an effective surrogate of risk of later atherosclerosis in the heart and brain causing heart attacks and strokes. Worldwide, the market for statins exceeds $20 billion. The strategy is appealing: patients at high risk are identified by their cholesterol level. They are given a statin and the serum cholesterol measured a month later. The patient and the doctor are both happy because they can see the potential long-term benefit through this surrogate measurement. But for cancer risk, we have nothing to measure as yet. However, it will come within the next 10 years for some types of cancer. Once we find biomarkers of risk then it becomes easy to motivate people to reduce that risk. Motivation creates compliance that in turn creates markets for products and services to drive the future. Of course it would be a move away from the current "wonder drug blockbuster" concept but it is inevitable over a 20-year timeframe.

Current cancer incidence figures demonstrate real health inequality: the percentage of smokers in the higher socio-economic classes is in low single figures, while the percentage in the lowest classes is still about 50% in parts of the UK. Despite the known risks of smoking, if friends and family smoke then there is little social pressure to stop. Banning smoking in public places will probably lead to a further drop of about 4%. Increases in tax have been a powerful disincentive to smoke but the price of a packet of cigarettes is now so high that smokers are turning to the black market. Lung cancer is a rare disease in higher socio-economic groups and now a disease associated with poverty.

Cancer genetics

The future prevention picture will be coloured by post-genomic research – research made possible as a result of mapping the human genome. Currently about 100 genes are associated with the development of a whole range of cancers. Carrying a changed version of a particular gene – or combination of changed genes – will not necessarily lead to the development of that cancer but will enable an individual to know whether or not they have increased risk.

Within 20 years most people in the developed world will be genetically mapped. The information – gained from a simple blood test – will be easily stored on a smart-card. Legislation will be required to prevent this information being used to determine an individual's future health status for mortgage, insurance, and employment purposes. However, the process of mapping will reveal that every person who has been screened will carry a predisposition to certain diseases. It will be an integral part of the process that unearthing a predisposition will bring advantages – not a prediction that the disease will necessarily develop. People will learn to live with risk. Possession of a particular gene will give the client and health professionals crucial intelligence. It might be important for the patient to be screened regularly in order to detect pre-cancerous cellular changes; or the client may be offered specific lifestyle advice on how to prevent the disease developing. If a cancer does develop, the genetic profile of that patient will help determine the best course of treatment.

The average age of diagnosis of cancer in Britain is 68. By 2020, improvements in screening, detection, and diagnosis will reduce this. A predisposition for some cancers, that used to manifest themselves in a patient's 70s or 80s, will be found in young adult life and detected and corrected successfully in the patient's 30s. Increasing age will remain the strongest risk predictor. Nevertheless, these techniques do raise the unwelcome spectre of individuals being told that they are among the 50% of the population who are not at risk of lung cancer if they smoke – although they may not be immune from a whole range of other chronic conditions.

Much of all this is already happening in some form but the computing power of the future will bring accurate calculation of risk and so individual predictions will take place on an unimaginable scale. Screening programmes will be developed on a national basis if they are simple, robust and cheap. Patients will expect the screening to take place at a convenient venue for them – the local pharmacy or health centre, for example, and not be painful or overly time-consuming. Health professionals, as well as consumers, will demand that any programme is accurate and does not give misleading results, and governments will demand that its cost will lead to more effective use of other resources. Novel providers of risk assessment services are likely to emerge.

REFERENCES

1. US Dept of Health and Human Services (1989) Reducing the health consequences of smoking. US Dept of Health and Human Services.
2. Scheu M. et al. (2004) The effects of a major cigarette price change on smoking behaviour in California: a zero-inflated negative binomial model. *Health Economics* 13: 781–791.
3. Wanless D. Securing Good Health for the Whole Population. UK Treasury 2004.
4. Bosanquet N. and Trigg A. (1991) A Smoke free Europe in the year 2000. In: *Wishful Thinking or Realistic Strategy?* Carden Publications. Chichester.
5. Bosanquet N. and Magee J. (1999) Adolescents and smoking; evidence from France and Spain. *Journal of Adolescence* 22: 601–605.
6. US Department of Health and Human Services (2004) Women, Tobacco and Cancer: An Agenda for the 21st century. US Dept of Health and Human Services.
7. Spooner A. (2004) Quality in the new GP Contract. Radcliffe Medical press.
8. Hung H. et al. (2004) Fruit and vegetable intake and risk of major chronic disease. *Journal of the National Cancer Institute* 96(21): 1577–1584.
9. Key T.J. (2004) Diet nutrition and the prevention of cancer. *Public Health Nutrition* 7(1A): 187–200.

3

Screening

Introduction

Cancer screening is one of the great controversies of modern medicine. The controversy is bound to increase as our knowledge of genetics improves. At the interface between public health and specialist care, its economics creates tensions between professional groups, politicians and the public: a screening test may be cheap, but applying it to a population (with rigorous quality control and effective processing of patients with abnormal results) creates a large workload and therefore sizeable cost. Screening can also have profound psychological effects on individuals with false-positive results who require investigation but are eventually found not to have cancer. Unless screening can be shown to reduce mortality rates from a specific cancer, the money used is often better spent on improving care, and this has led to a disparity in screening recommendations between countries. The human genome project is likely to provide new approaches to cancer-risk assessment and will bring new challenges to this complex area.

There is a contrast between extensive and largely uncritical public support for screening, and the very real difficulties in organising effective programmes. There has been one great success – cervical cancer screening on a population basis. This programme has been able to reduce incidence and mortality in some developed countries with particular success in the UK and Scandinavia. In addition, there has been some success from mammography programmes. The balance of evidence suggests that screening for breast cancer has had positive results; perhaps most of all through a general stirring up effect that has encouraged improvements in early detection and staging. Screening for colo-rectal cancer is confined to the USA and it will be 10 years before we know whether trial results can be turned into effective population-based screening programmes. Screening detects less than 15%

of all new cases worldwide and less than 10% of cancers in developed countries, excluding colo-rectal cancer. Thus it would be wrong to neglect screening. However, it would also be wrong to ignore how selective it is, and that considerable investment in time and resources is required to start successful programmes. Screening is not a magic solution or an easy option and least of all in less developed countries where there has been little success in developing low-cost screening programmes.

Cancer screening is defined as the systematic application of a test to individuals who have not sought medical attention because of symptoms. It may be opportunistic (offered to patients consulting their doctor for another reason) or population-based (covering a predefined age range, with elaborate call and recall systems). The risk of dying from a cancer increases with the stage at which it is diagnosed and so the degree at which it has spread. The aim of screening is to detect cancer in its early, asymptomatic phase. The problem is that many screening tests are relatively crude, and cancers may have metastasised even in an effective screening programme before they are detected.

False positives

Sensitivity varies between tests. A 100% sensitive test detects all cancers in the screened population. The most rigorous means of calculating sensitivity is to determine the proportion of expected cancers not presenting as interval cases between screens. Good cancer registration is essential when making this calculation. Specificity is the proportion of negative results produced by a test in individuals without cancer. A 100% specific test gives no false-positive results. Investigation of patients without cancer is a major factor in the cost of screening.

Bias

The advantages and disadvantages of screening must be considered carefully: they will vary between cancers and tests. The three main problems in assessing the benefit of any screening test for cancer are: lead-time bias, length bias and selection bias, all of which impair the effectiveness of screening as a method of reducing cancer mortality. *Lead-time bias* advances the diagnosis but does not prolong survival: as occurs when the disease has already metastasised even though the primary tumour is still small, patients die at the same time as if the disease had not been detected early.

Length bias results in diagnosis of less aggressive tumours. Rapidly grow-ing cancers, which generally have a poor prognosis, present in the screening interval thereby reducing the value of the screening process. *Selection bias* occurs even in the most well-organised health care systems: worried but healthy individuals (who would present with cancer symptoms early) com-ply with screening, whereas less well-educated and socially disadvantaged individuals do not. In the UK, the National health services (NHS's) breast cancer-screening programme compliance rates vary widely between com-munities depending on their relative deprivation.

Rational decision-making about cancer screening requires a detailed analysis of factors that may vary between populations:

- *The cancer should be common* and its natural history should be properly understood. This allows a realistic prediction of the proposed test's likely value.
- *The test should be effective (high sensitivity and specificity)* and should be acceptable to the population. Cervical smears, for example, are difficult to perform in many Islamic countries where women prefer not to undergo vaginal examination, and the take-up rate for colonoscopy is low in asymp-tomatic individuals because it is uncomfortable and sometimes unpleasant.
- *The health care system must be able to cope* with patients who produce posi-tive results and require investigation. This may be a particular problem at the start of a population-based study.
- Ultimately, *screening must improve the survival rate* in a randomised-controlled setting.

The natural history of many cancers (including incidence and mortality) may change over time for reasons that are poorly understood. In Europe, the incidence of stomach cancer has decreased dramatically over the last few decades, whereas deaths from breast cancer reached a peak in the UK in 1989 and have decreased slightly each year since.

Lobby groups often exercise political pressure to implement screening programmes (even when their effectiveness is undemonstrated), and manu-facturers of equipment or suppliers of reagents may exercise commercial pressure. In "fee-for-service-based" provider systems, there is a financial inducement for doctors to screen and investigate because doing nothing earns no money. The launch of the NHS breast screening service by the UK government in 1989 was viewed by many as a pre-election vote-winning exercise rather than a rational public health intervention even though it now commands general support. There are now similar pressures to introduce prostate cancer screening, though uncertainty remains about the management of men with slightly elevated prostate-specific antigen (PSA).

The ultimate measure of success in a screening programme is a demonstrable reduction in mortality in the screened population. However, this needs large numbers of individuals, and at least 10-year assessment in most of the common cancers. Although randomised studies may show conclusive benefit, it must be remembered that the expertise and professional enthusiasm available to a study population may be considerably greater than that achievable under subsequent field conditions. Quality of mammography interpretation and investigation of breast abnormalities are good examples of this, and may explain the relatively patchy results of breast screening in practice across Europe. Case-control studies using age-matched individuals from the same population and non-randomised comparison between areas providing and not providing screening may give useful indicators, but are not as conclusive as randomised trials. Surrogate measures of effectiveness can be used to assess a programme with relatively small numbers of patients soon after its implementation, but are insufficient to prove that screening saves lives:

- When a population is first screened, a higher than expected incidence of cancer should be seen because screening is detecting cancer that would not present with symptoms for several years.
- Tumour down-staging is a second measure of impact. An increase in early-stage cancer detection and, consequently, reduction in advanced disease are expected over 3–5 years.
- The third, short-term evaluation is a comparison of the survival of screen-detected patients with that of those presenting symptomatically.

Success in terms of these three indices may not necessarily be translated into a useful screening programme. In the 1970s, a study of routine chest radiography and sputum cytology to detect lung cancer showed a 5-year survival of 40% in screen-detected patients, compared with an overall figure of 5%, but a reduction in mortality from lung cancer has not been achieved. For most types of screening there will be quite substantial increases in treatment required as incidence increases.

We review the evidence below both on the impact on treatment and on cost. Screening will also have a major impact on requirement for diagnostics

> **Box 3.1: Assessing cancer risk**
> 1. It will be possible for an individual's genome to be sequenced in a day.
> 2. Much more precision in predictive statements about risk will be possible.
> 3. Personalised medicine will be in part based on genetic background.
> 4. Enhanced screening will be offered to those with pre-malignant molecular changes.
> 5. We may have a molecular rheostat for cancer read by an implanted chip.
> 6. Effective prevention strategies will stimulate better risk assessment.
> 7. Better health education will be a key component in the use of screening.

and may have perverse effects in slowing down access by patients with urgent problems who have not been referred as a result of screening but through other routes. Thus screening programmes may have unwanted side effects.

In addition to its past difficult history a range of new issues and decisions is about to emerge in cancer screening, leading to profound ethical, educational, commercial and medical challenges. Completion of the human genome project, and the ability to handle large volumes of sequence data and assay for mutations rapidly and cheaply using gene chip technology, will raise potential for cancer-risk assessment (Box 3.1). Commercial pressures have led the major pharmaceutical companies to invest heavily in genomics: their interest is to discover new drugs and to tailor therapies more specifically to individual patients. It is likely that groups of individuals with no family history of cancer will be identified as being at significantly increased risk of developing cancer. Devising optimal screening schedules for such groups will be a major challenge. The technology of screening will also change. Within 10 years, it may become feasible to implant into the body a sophisticated gene chip that continually monitors for specific DNA changes: when these are found, a warning signal would be transmitted to the domestic information technology system and an appropriate appointment made at the local clinic. The type of therapy given will depend as much on genetic changes in the tumour cell as on the tumour type itself.

Cervical cancer

The Papanicolaou (Pap) test is the test most commonly used for cervical cancer screening. It involves taking a sample of cells from the exocervix, the transformation zone, and the endocervix using a flat wooden spatula. The cells are then transferred onto a glass slide and fixed using an alcohol-based solution. The slides are then stained at the laboratory and are read by cyto-screeners and cytologists.

Liquid-based cytology (LBC) is an alternative method that is being adopted by several countries. It has been developed with the aim of reducing the unsatisfactory rate and reducing the number of false-negative slides. After collecting the cells from the cervix, they are transferred straight into a vial containing preservation fluid. The suspension of cells within in the vial is then used to create a monolayer of cells on a slide. We review here the experience of three countries: the UK, Australia and Finland, which have organised screening programmes, comparing their experience with three countries that have opportunistic screening: the USA, France and Germany.

The United Kingdom

The Pap test is currently being used throughout England and Wales, while LBC is used in Scotland. Both England and Wales are planning to implement LBC in the near future. Cervical cancer screening, using the Pap test, began in the mid-1960s in the UK. By the mid-1980s, many women were having regular smear tests. However, concern was raised that many of the women who were at the greatest risk of developing cervical cancer had never undergone a smear test. With a view to eradicating this problem, the NHS Cervical Screening Programme was established in 1988.

Local health authorities introduced computerised call–recall systems and were instructed to meet certain quality standards. Under the national programme, women aged between 25 and 64 years are eligible for a smear test once every 3–5 years. Depending on the result of the test, they will either be invited for a repeat smear in 3–5 years (a negative result), a repeat smear in 6 months (borderline) or referred to colposcopy for further investigation (cellular abnormalities present).

Currently, approximately 13.8 million women are eligible for screening; 81.6% of eligible women in 2000/2001 had had a smear test in the previous 5 years. In England, the screening programme cost approximately £150 million per year. This equates to a cost of about £37.50 for each smear test.

The incidence of and mortality from cervical cancer have decreased in the UK by more than 40% since the introduction of the screening programme. However, such calculations underestimate the full effect of the screening programme, as cervical cancer mortality might have continued to rise, which is what happened from 1967 to 1987:

Cervical cancer mortality in England and Wales in women younger than 35 years rose threefold from 1967 to 1987. By 1988, incidence in this age-range was among the highest in the world despite substantial opportunistic screening. Since national screening was started in 1988, this rising trend has been reversed. Cervical screening has prevented an epidemic that would have killed one in 65 of all British women born since 1950 and culminated in about 6000 deaths per year.[1]

Australia

Opportunistic screening was first introduced in the 1960s. In 1991, a national screening programme was established as a joint initiative of the Commonwealth, the State and the Territory Governments.

All women aged 20–70 years should be screened once every 2 years using the Pap test. Between January 2000 and December 2001, 61.8% of the target population were screened. The following table represents the participation in the screening population by age for this time period.

Age	20–24	25–29	30–34	35–39	40–44	45–49	50–54	55–59	60–64	65–69
Participation (%)	50.3	61.4	64.9	67.1	68.1	67.4	70.2	62.1	55.7	45.3

The recruitment of women to the screening programme is done at a state or territory level. Women from particular groups associated with lower attendance rates such as older women or aboriginal women are targeted more aggressively. The screening programme has resulted in a reduction in the mortality of women due to cervical cancer. In 1982, the age-standardised mortality for women aged 20–69 years was 5.1 per 100,000 women. In 2001, this figure fell to 2.4 per 100,000 women. The service is free to all eligible women in Australia.

Finland

Organised cervical screening was introduced in the early 1960s. By 1970, the coverage of the invitational programme was already above 80% of women in the target age group. Women aged 30–60 years are targeted. Current policy states that they should be offered screening using the Pap test once every 5 years (if their results are normal). The coverage of invitations sent to the eligible population in 1996 was 89.5%. According to information from an annual population survey, the proportion of all Pap smears (including both opportunistic and diagnostic smears in addition to the programme smears), taken during a 5-year period was approximately 93% for women in the target age group. The coverage of any smears during a lifetime was 98%.[2]

During 1955–1964, the incidence of invasive cervical cancer in Finland was 15 cases per 100,000 woman-years (age-adjusted to the world standard population) with a slight increasing trend within that period. During the years 1991–1995, the incidence rates varied from 2.8 to 4.5 cases per 100,000 woman-years, indicating an overall decrease of approximately 70–80% in the age-adjusted rate. Mortality from cervical cancer was approximately seven cases per 100,000 woman-years from 1955 to 1964. The age-adjusted mortality rate in 1995 was 0.8 cases per 100,000 woman-years.

The direct screening cost for the municipalities, including the costs for invitational material and other printed material, mailing, sample-taking supplies, sample-staining and analysis, informing the women, and registration has been in the order of approximately 10 ECU per smear. The organised programme has been very cheap and has led to positive net savings when compared with its cost-effectiveness. Later reviews are even more positive:

In Finland the organised screening programme for the prevention of cervical cancer has been run for over 30 years and has contributed to a 70–80% decrease in the age-adjusted cervical cancer incidence, as well as a reduction in mortality rates.[3]

The screening programme is estimated to have avoided more than 200 deaths a year from cervical cancer. There is a 90% coverage of the 30–60 age groups with screening every 5 years.

France

In France, prior to 1990 there was no organised mass-screening programme, but opportunistic screening had already become fairly widespread, correlating with the appearance in the 1960s of oral and intra-uterine contraceptives. At present, six million cervical smears are taken each year, mostly by gynaecologists. This number is large enough to offer a good coverage of the target population. However, 40% of the French women have never had a cervical smear test. This rate increases up to 50% in women older than 55 years and 80% after the age of 60 years. In contrast, most women under 55 years have a cytological test annually.

The intervention procedures for cervical cancer screening were defined at a consensus conference held in Lille in 1990. The major recommendations were to screen all women, exclusively by cervical smears, in the age group 25–65 years, every 3 years following two negative smears. Since 1990, organised programmes have been implemented in various areas (Departments) of France. The success of these programmes has varied. The coverage achieved in each region was monitored: this ranged from approximately 20% to 80%. The age of participants was an important factor with the participation being much higher for the younger generation. The rate of abnormal tests varied from 0.2% to 3% while the detection of cancer ranged from 0.04% to 0.15%. In November 1998 a law was passed stating that the smear test will be offered free of charge to eligible women in France.[4]

There is currently little data available on the cost of the cervical cancer-screening programme in France. However, general statements can be made. The screening programme is decentralised which makes it a much more costly service to run than that in many other European countries in which a centralised model has been adopted. If the participation rate were to be increased, it is likely that the overall cost of running the programme would be reduced.[5]

Germany

The Pap test was first introduced in West Germany in the 1950s. In 1971, the national screening programme was established. This led to the entitlement of all women covered by statutory health insurance (greater than 90% of female population) to a free annual smear test. After the re-unification of East and West Germany in 1991 the national screening programme was extended to all women in East Germany. (Twenty-five million insurees in West Germany and 5.5 million in East Germany eligible to attend the screening programme.)

The current policy is that all women aged 20 years and older are eligible to attend a smear test annually. No upper age limit has been stipulated. In any given year, more than half the women attending screening observe a 1-year screening interval. Attendance rates over a 3-year period currently exceed 80% of the eligible female population. In recent years, the attendance rate in West Germany has been slightly higher than in East Germany. A region in

West Germany for which there is data available concerning the incidence of cancer is Saarland. In this region, the age-standardised incidence of invasive cancer decreased by more than 50% in the decade following the introduction of the national screening programme (from 29.2 per 100,000 in 1970–1972 to 13 per 100,000 in 1979–1981, world standard). The available data for the subsequent time period show a slight but steady decline in both regions of the country, down to 11 per 100,000 in 1988–1990 in Saarland, and 21 per 100,000 in East Germany. Age-standardised mortality rates of cervical cancer decreased by approximately one-third in Saarland and East Germany during the 1970s (Saarland: from 7 per 100,000 in 1970–1972 to 4 per 100,000 in 1979–1981; East Germany: from 11 per 100,000 in 1970–1972 to 7 per 100,000 in 1979–1981, world standard). The reduction in mortality rates in both parts of the country was approximately 20% during the 1980s. Based on estimates of all available data from other regions of the country, the overall cervical cancer mortality in West Germany has decreased from 6 per 100,000 in 1970–1972 to 3 per 100,000 in 1988–1990.

In contrast with the sharp decline in the incidence of invasive cervical cancer, the incidence of cervical carcinoma *in situ* increased sharply in the Saarland shortly after the introduction of the national screening programme (from 12 per 100,000 in 1970–1972 to 20 per 100,000 in 1973–1975). By the end of the 1970s, the incidence of cervical carcinoma had fallen slightly below the level at the beginning of the decade (10 per 100,000 in 1979–1981, world standard). Subsequently, the age-standardised incidence declined gradually to 8 per 100,000 in 1988–1990. In contrast, the age-standardised incidence of cervical *in situ* carcinoma increased steadily in East Germany during the 1970s (from 30 per 100,000 in 1970–1972 to 42 per 100,000 in 1979–1981, world standard). In the latter half of the 1980s, the incidence of cervical *in situ* cancer in East Germany stabilised at 41 per 100,000 (1988–1989, world standard).

Approximately 90% of the cervical cancer-screening examinations are performed by office-based gynaecologists (10% by general practitioners) who receive a fee standardised on a national floating point scale, the monetary value of which depends on regional contracts negotiated between the regional association of office-based physicians and insurance funds. No remuneration is provided for smears that are unsatisfactory for cytological examination. As a result, the number of smears classified as unsatisfactory is very low.[6]

United States of America

The USA reported the highest rates of testing for cervical cancer in the world with 88.0% of women aged 18–64 years reporting a Pap test within the previous 3 years and 77.3% even among those with no health insurance. This was mainly based on opportunistic screening and did not have results for incidence and mortality (3.3 per 100,000), which were better than the UK (3.9) or Finland (1.3). It would appear that the USA system had achieved wide coverage but at a high cost and possibly with too great a frequency. The American Cancer Society's screening guidelines were hard to reconcile with the age groups used in European screening programmes:

Screening should begin approximately 3 years after a woman begins having vaginal intercourse but no later than 21 years of age. Screening should be done every year with regular Pap tests or every 2 years using liquid-based tests. At or after the age of 30, women who have had three normal test results in a row may get screened every 2–3 years.[7]

Screening can stop at age 70. Thus a woman in the USA might be screened some 50 times compared to 10 times in the UK.

In order to increase the participation of women with little or no health insurance, The National Breast and Cervical Cancer Early Detection Programme (NBCCEDP) was established in 1991. It was implemented with a view to offer screening programmes to women with low incomes and to those who are either underinsured or underserved. It is present in all 50 states. It entitles women aged 18+ to free cervical screening (using the Pap test) at least once every 3 years. To date, 1.9 million women have been screened on one of the programmes (4.6 million screening examinations have been carried out). The programme received $210 million in 2004. This is used for the running of Pap tests, diagnostic testing for women with an abnormal test, surgical consultations, as well as mammograms and clinical breast examinations.

Each state receives funds that are to be used to create and distribute educational resources to women, especially targeting those who have never been screened or are infrequent attendees. NBCCEDP assures that the same quality of service is provided throughout the country as a whole.

Breast cancer screening

The method used to detect breast cancer is mammography. This involves X-raying each of the breasts in turn to look for small changes within the breast.

Table 3.1.

Country	Programme type	Year programme began	Detection methods	Age groups covered by mammography	Screening interval (40–49)	Screening interval (50+)
Denmark	SPR	1991	MM	50–69	NA	2
France	NR	1989	MM, CBE	50–74	NA	2
Iceland	N	1987	MM, CBE	40–69	2	2
Italy	NR	2000	MM	50–69	NA	2
Luxembourg	N	1992	MM	50–69	NA	2
Netherlands	N	1989	MM	50–74	NA	2
Norway	N	1996	MM	50–69	NA	2
Portugal	SPR	1990	MM, CBE, BSE	45–64	2	2
Spain	SPR	1990	MM	45–69	2	2
Sweden	SPR	1986	MM	40–74[2]	1.7	2
Finland	N	1989	MM	50–59	NA	2–3
Switzerland	SPR	1999	MM	50–69	NA	2
UK	N	1988	MM	50–64	NA	3
Canada	NR	1988	MM, CBE[1]	50–69	NA	2
US	MMRS	1995	MM, CBE	40+	1–2	1–2
Australia	NR	1991	MM	50–69	NA	2
Japan	N	2002	MM, CBE	50–69	NA	2
New Zealand	N	1998	MM	50–64	NA	2

SPR: state/provincial/regional; NR: national with regional implementation; N: national; MMRS: Mammography registry system; MM: mammography; CBE: clinical breast examination; BSE: breast self-examination; 1: in 5 of the 12 programmes; 2: in half of the counties the lower age is 40; in the other half it is 50. International Breast Screening Network: characteristics of breast screening programmes: responses to survey in 2002.

The breast is compressed as this decreases the dose of radiation received by the woman. As a person's age increases, the glandular tissue within the breast is gradually replaced by fat. Fatty tissue is less dense therefore the resulting images are of a higher quality. Furthermore, glandular tissue has a higher risk of radiation-induced carcinogenisis thus younger women are not routinely screened.

This technique allows the detection of small changes in the tissue therefore it is possible to identify cancers which are too small to be felt or seen by either the patient or the doctor.

United Kingdom

An organised screening programme (the first of its kind) was implemented in 1988. Women were first invited in 1990. By the mid-1990s, national coverage was achieved. Women aged 50–64 years are currently invited to attend a screening test every 3 years. Work is being done to extend this to women aged 70 years. This should be fully in place by the end of 2004. A further change is that two views will be taken of the breast at each screening instead of simply the first as this has been shown to increase the detection of cancer by as much as 43%.[8] Women whom are older than 64 and close to 70 are encouraged to arrange their own appointment. Approximately 1.5 million women are screened (free of charge to them) each year. Screening takes place in a number of environments, including hospitals, permanent convenient locations (e.g. shopping centres) and mobile centres. In 1998/1989, 110,000 women accepted screening invitations. This increased dramatically to 1.5 million in 2002/2003.[9]

A report published in 2000 demonstrated that mortality rates associated with breast cancer had reduced for 55–69-year olds. It was estimated that at least 300 lives are being saved each year as a result of the programme. This is predicted to increase to 1250 lives per year by 2010.[10] Mortality rates in 1999 were 20% less than those in the mid-1980s.

The current budget for the screening programme (including the actual cost of screening) is approximately £52 million. This equates to ~£30 per woman invited or ~£40 per woman screened. To date over 14 million women have been screened within the programme. This has led to the detection of more than 80,000 cancers.

However there are some differences between the short-run estimates from the screening programmes and the long-term changes in survival. For the USA, which has the best data on longer-term survival, there was little difference in improved survival between patients with breast cancer and patients with types of cancer such as kidney and colo-rectal where screening was either non-existent or with very low coverage. The main reasons for the definite improvement would appear to be better access to chemotherapy rather than screening.

Australia

Breast screening began on a national basis in Australia in 1991 (it has been called BreastScreen Australia since 1994). In 1990, the Commonwealth announced funding of $64 million over 3 years to implement a national program for the early detection of breast cancer, based on the recommendations in the Screening Evaluation Co-ordination Unit report. The programme offers a free mammogram once every 2 years to eligible women. Those aged 50–69 years are targeted. They are required to book their own appointment but are sent reminders. Those aged 70+ are still eligible for screening but are not sent reminders. Two views of the breast are taken at each screening.

The programme is funded by the Commonwealth and each of the State and Territory Governments. It is administered via State Coordination Units. There are more than 500 locations at which screening can be conducted. These range from fixed, relocatable and mobile screening units and cover urban, rural and remote areas. The State and Territory Governments have primary responsibility for the implementation of "BreastScreen" at a local level while the Commonwealth oversees the entire programme (i.e. ensure consistent standards across states, collect data and monitor results).[11]

In 2000–2001 time period, 1.6 million women were screened, 98% of whom were aged between 50 and 69 years; 57% of women aged 50–69 years in Australia took part in the program during these 2 years. This had been rising steadily over recent years (51.4% for 1996–1997 and 55.6% for 1999–2000). The participation in the different states can be seen below.

	Australia	New South Wales	Victoria	Queensland	West Australia	South Australia	Tasmania	Northern Territory	Australian Capital Territory
Rate (%)	56.9	53.0	59.2	58.4	55.4	64.3	60.0	46.3	57.0

There was little difference in participation rates for different social classes. However, rates were significantly lower for indigenous women (36.2%).[12] During the time period 2000–2001, 43 cancers were detected per 10,000 women screened, 28 of which were small cancers. The proportion of women recalled for assessment because of an abnormal mammogram result was significantly higher for women being screened for the first time in 2001 compared with women who had previously been screened. The age-standardised recall rate was 8.3% for women attending their first round of screening. For women attending their second or subsequent screen, only 4.0% (age-standardised) were recalled for assessment because of an abnormal result.[13]

Effect of screening on incidence and mortality.
Aged 50–69

	1987	2000
Incidence (per 100,000 women)	197.1	269.9
Mortality (per 100,000 women)	66.8	51.8

Australia's National Cancer Prevention Policy 06/2004.

A similar pattern can be seen for women aged 70+ while for women younger than 50, mortality has consistently been less than eight per 100,000 women. Improvements have been made in the years since introducing BreastScreen. The following table displays the number of deaths from breast cancer per 100,000 women for the whole of Australia.[14]

	1993	1994	1995	1996	1997	1998	% change between 1993 and 1998
All ages	26.9	26.5	25.6	25.0	24.2	23.0	−14.9
<50	6.4	6.6	5.8	6.3	6.4	5.8	−4.3
50–69	71.5	68.6	68.5	65.0	62.8	59.4	−16.9

National Information Report 1999/2000. Public Health Outcome by the Department of Health and Ageing.

United States of America

The survival rate 5 years after diagnosis of breast cancer increased from 72.3% between 1982 and 1986 to 84.0% between 1992 and 1997. These encouraging results can be attributed to early detection through screening combined with improvements in treatment and drug therapies. There is little information on the cost of the screening programme though a figure of $100 per screen has been suggested.

The NBCCEDP, described earlier in the section referring to cervical cancer screening, offers free mammograms to underinsured women from aged 40 onwards in an attempt to increase the participation rates.

Table 3.2 displays the death rates for breast cancer for females in the USA for the time period 1950–2001. (Deaths per 100,000 of population.)

Table 3.2. Death rates for breast cancer per 100,000 Population in US females from 1950–2001.

	1950	1960	1970	1980	1990	1995	2000	2001
All ages (age-adjusted)	31.9	31.7	32.1	31.9	33.3	30.5	26.8	26.0
All ages (crude)	24.7	26.1	28.4	30.6	34.0	32.2	29.2	28.6
Under 25	–	–	–	–	–	–	–	–
25–34	3.8	3.8	3.9	3.3	2.9	2.6	2.3	2.4
35–44	20.8	20.2	20.4	17.9	17.8	14.9	12.4	12.4
45–54	46.9	51.4	52.6	48.1	45.4	41.0	33.0	32.8
55–64	69.9	70.8	77.6	80.5	78.6	69.4	59.3	57.5
65–74	95.0	90.0	93.8	101.1	111.7	102.8	88.3	85.8
75–84	139.8	129.9	127.4	126.4	146.3	140.1	128.9	125.8
85+	195.5	191.9	157.1	169.3	196.3	200.2	205.7	188.9

For countries that have developed screening programmes there is a strong commitment to mammography. However, results have not been as strong as in screening for cervical cancer, which can be turned into a rare disease for women under 60. Mammography contributes to early detection and may have a halo effect according to the leader or czar of the UK cancer programme in encouraging better and quicker service:

I have a hunch that the breast screening programme has a halo effect around it so that by the very fact that you have a screening service you improve all the other services.[15]

The screening programme contributes to earlier detection although even where it exists more than half of cancers diagnosed are either from people who have been diagnosed in the interval between mammographies or those who have not been screened at all. One of the most detailed and careful studies was carried out in Tilburg in the Netherlands where it was possible to follow up a large population before and after the introduction of screening. Among women in the screened population 50–69 the proportion of early-stage cancers rose from 24% to 45% while there was no significant changes in staging for the under 50 or over 70 age groups. The study concludes both on a positive no end with an appropriate note of caution:

In conclusion, improved prognosis and a more favourable breast carcinoma stage distribution were observed among patient ages 50–69 years during the period 1992–1999.

In this age group, patients with screen-detected tumours had a better prognosis than did patients with interval or clinically-detected malignancies. Whether this improved prognosis and earlier diagnosis will result in substantial reduction in breast carcinoma mortality remains to be seen. Even after the full implementation of the screening programme in 1996, the majority of invasive malignancies were still detected between screening rounds or in patients who did not participate in the programme.[16]

A long-term study in Finland showed that recurrence as well as survival was improved from screening. Women identified from the Finnish cancer registry as having breast cancer in 1991 and 1992 were followed up. The median follow-up time was 9.5 years. Women with cancers detected through screening had better survival and less recurrence even for tumours of similar size.[17]

Colo-rectal cancer screening

The main experience with colo-rectal cancer screening has been in the USA. The strength of public support for screening in general has been very supportive. The United States Preventive Task Force strongly recommends that "clinicians screen men and women 50 years of age or older for colo-rectal cancer". However, the detailed review of the evidence in the report was difficult to fit to such a strong recommendation:

The USPSTF found fair to good evidence that periodic fecal occult blood testing (FOBT) reduces mortality from colo-rectal cancer and fair evidence that sigmoido-scopy alone or in combination with FOBT reduces mortality. The USPTF did not find direct evidence that screening colonoscopy is effective in reducing colo-rectal cancer mortality …

There are insufficient data to determine which strategy is best in terms of the balance of benefits and potential harms or cost-effectiveness. Studies reviewed by the USPSTF indicate that colo-rectal cancer screening is likely to be most effective (less than $30,000 per additional life year gained) regardless of the strategy chosen.[18]

The international evidence on the impact of screening is also available. Based on comparisons from the WHO for the USA from 1985–1995, the incidence of colo-rectal cancer fell, while in Australia and Denmark it rose.

It is possible that increased screening was part of the reason for this change. The World Cancer Report sums up the position well:

Some health authorities in developed countries acknowledge the legitimacy of a screening protocol for colo-rectal cancer. However, the high cost of a generalised intervention and the limited acceptance of the tests by the population explain its limited application.[19]

A pilot programme in the UK covered two areas of England and Scotland. The aim was to examine whether FOBT could be used as a screening technique with results for populations, which were as good as the earlier trial. The take-up rate was 59% overall but much lower among certain groups – for example 33% among males in deprived areas. The cost per quality adjusted life year (QALY) was positive:

Our model suggests that over the expected lifetime for a 50-year-old male, the estimated net cost per QALY gained is around £2,600. While there is no official cut-off for a societal willingness to pay for a QALY, National institute for clinical excellence (NICE) has recommended technologies that have a net cost of around £30,000 per QALY gained.[20]

The main problem seen for any extension is the likely workload for secondary care:

Our data suggest that at least one additional colonoscopy session for every dedicated screening session might be required in the first 5 years of the programme, with requirements increasing after that due to a cumulative effect. There will also be a need for additional consultant sessions for dealing with pathology.[20]

It would be likely to take several years for additional investment in capacity and there would then be several years before full coverage of the UK population would be reached. The UK was moving forward but there was little sign that the oldest screening services in Scandinavia were following.

Some of the most long-term experience with colo-rectal cancer screening was found with health care maintenance organisations (HMOs) on the American West Coast. The Group health Co-operative of Washington State carried out a retrospective study of cancers diagnosed from 1993 to 1999. During this time, 206 cancers were detected by screening and 717 by symptoms. In the 3 months before diagnosis, costs were significantly lower for screen-detected cancer as were treatment costs in the first 12 months. Overall costs were 32.9% lower for patients with screen-detected cancers: $29,921 compared to $39,513. If such results were repeated more widely they would greatly alter the cost-effectiveness profile for colo-rectal cancer screening.[21]

Colo-rectal cancer screening could have particular relevance in central Europe where diet and other factors may be affecting the cancer rate. Using data from the National Health Insurance Fund of Hungary, Boncz and colleagues have estimated results for screening in Hungary. The cost of treatment of colo-rectal cancer in Hungary in 2001 was $34.8 million. In the age group 45–65 years (with a 10% mortality decline), 718 lives could be saved, and with a 20% mortality decline 1462 lives could be saved during a 10-year screening programme. The cost per life year saved varied from $1074 to $4381 depending on the mortality decline and the screening strategy.[22]

Prostate cancer: In the USA and much of Europe, the prevalence of prostate cancer has increased by more than 100% in the last 10 years. Greater longevity is partly responsible, but the principal reason for this increase is earlier detection using serum PSA testing. Post-mortem examinations of men over 70 years of age have consistently shown a prevalence of prostate cancer of more than 50%. Thus, when PSA screening is introduced in an asymptomatic population the reported incidence increases dramatically.

Several techniques are being developed to improve the performance of the PSA assay in distinguishing aggressive from indolent cancer. These include use of free and complexed PSA ratios, PSA density (relating serum PSA level to gland volume), aged-adjusted PSA rate of increase of PSA, and variation in the cut-off level. As holistic genomic and proeomic methods become more widely used, it is likely that improved understanding of the natural history of the disease in an individual will lead to more personalised therapy following needle biopsy to access tissue.

The best treatment for screen-detected patients has not been determined. Many die of another condition with no morbidity caused by their prostate disease. Localised prostate cancer can be managed by radical surgery or radiotherapy, or by doing nothing. Younger patients favour more active treatment but must cope with the side effects, which include incontinence, impotence, strictures and disordered bowel habit that often persists for many years. A large, population-based study from the USA has shown no survival advantage after 11 years in men offered intensive screening. A recent authoritative review by the UK Department of Health concluded that there is no place for screening programmes at present, but that there is a need for a properly conducted randomised trial. Current UK practice is to offer screening only to men over 50 years of age who have been given reliable information about its benefits and hazards. PSA remains a useful investigation in men with symptoms of urinary outflow obstruction.

Conclusions

Screening was well supported by the public in the USA. A recent survey showed that 87% in a national telephone survey of 500 participants thought that routine cancer screening was almost always a good idea even if it revealed disease which could not be treated or which as likely to be asymptomatic (Table 3.3). Most would like to be screened by a whole body computerised tomography (CT) scan rather than to receive a cheque for $1000 even though such screening is actively discouraged by the American Society of Physicists in Medicine.[23] Very recently, however, the trend for people to pay for whole body CT scans has declined and some of the large businesses set up to sell up scanning to the general public are closing down. CT Screening International which in 2002 scanned 25,000 people at 13 centres across the USA has closed. These businesses used direct to consumer advertising suggesting that serious diseases could be discovered early but professional societies warned that the tests would mostly find innocuous abnormalities that would require extensive and sometimes painful, investigation.

Overall the costs of screening in the leading nation in screening programmes had risen to $10 billion (or 10% of total expenditures on the actual treatment of cancers). Much of the screening was for frequently repeated opportunities – screening which was not likely to be very effective – but the reach of screening in the USA health system was such that, 70–80% coverage was being achieved.

Outside the USA, there was agreement that the most cost-effective programmes were those that achieved full coverage with infrequent screening, but such programmes were very difficult to organise on a national basis. The gains to full coverage were set out in a study carried out for Denmark.[24] To illustrate: a screening programme that performs a test on the 20- to 69-year olds every third year but only has a participation rate of 70% will have the same amount of life years as a screening programme with a target group of 20- to 69-year olds, a screening interval of 4 years and a participation rate of 90%.

Table 3.3. General beliefs about early detection

	Respondents weighted % (N = 500)
How often does finding cancer early mean that treatment saves lives?	
None of the time	3
Some of the time	24
Most of the time	58
All of the time	16
How often does finding cancer early mean that a person can have less treatment?	
None of the time	3
Some of the time	44
Most of the time	42
All of the time	11
If there was a kind of cancer for which nothing can be done, would you want to be tested to see if you have it?	
Yes	66
No	34
Have you ever heard of cancers that grow so slowly that they are unlikely to cause you problems in your lifetime?	
Yes	52
No	48
Would you want to be tested to see if you had a slow-growing cancer like that?	
Yes	56
No	44
Routine screening means testing healthy persons to find cancer before they have any symptoms. Do you think routine cancer screening for healthy persons is almost always a good idea?	
Yes	87
No	13

Source: Schwartz et al., 2004.

There is however a great difference in costliness of these two programmes. The second programme is approximately 150 million DDK less expensive over a period of 36 years. It is clearly more cost-effective to improve participation rates than moving along the efficiency curve (extending the target group and/or reducing the screening interval). Could there be more cost-effective ways of achieving early detection? For cervical cancer the case for comprehensive screening programmes was a very strong one. For breast and colo-rectal cancers in systems where screening is not yet started fully, it would be better to start programmes on a city or regional basis. The population of Finland is about the same as that of a city region in nations with larger populations and would provide some guide to more local programmes. They could also target areas with particularly high incidence of specific cancers.

Outside the developed health systems the key screening priority was to develop targeted screening programmes in middle-income countries. There was little hope of starting screening programmes in low-income countries. One review sponsored by WHO concluded that:

Many low-income developing countries, particularly those in sub-Saharan Africa, currently have neither the financial and manpower resources nor the capacity in their health services to organise and sustain a screening programme of any sort.[25]

The feasible aim was to develop targeted programmes in middle-income countries. In the past, these programmes had covered wide age groups and carried out frequent screening, often with a low take-up rate. In Colombia (Mortality per 100,000 was 13.7 compared to 3.3 in the USA and 1.3 in Finland) and Mexico (17.1), quite wide opportunistic screening had little effect. However, in Chile (10.6), targeted screening programmes were successful in reducing death rates.[25]

There remained a contrast between the high profile of screening in health systems and their level of effectiveness. There had been a very real success in cervical cancer, and in breast cancer, screening had been a factor in raising survival rates from 70% to 90%: but this improvement in survival was found in all systems – in France and Italy as well as in the USA. For 1985–1989, the 5-year survival rate was 82.0% in France and 79.0% in Italy compared to 83.8% for the USA in a later period 1989–1995.

Another key area for research could be on methods of encouraging early detection by primary care physicians and specialists who might make initial referrals. One study in the UK showed how there could be substantial improvement in the accuracy of referral.[26] Even in areas with very successful screening programmes most patients with cancer would be unscreened, and overall, across all cancers the great majority of cancers would be unscreened. As they expanded, there was a danger that screening programmes would take time and resources away from other potential ways of encouraging early detection across the whole disparate field of cancer.

REFERENCES

1. Peto J. et al. (2004) The Cervical cancer epidemic that screening has prevented in the UK. *The Lancet* 364(9430): 249–256.
2. WHO. World Cancer Report. IARC, Lyon, 2003.
3. Anttila A. and Nieminen P. (2000) Cervical screening programme in Finland. *European Journal for Cancer* 36(17): 2209–2214.
4. Schaffer P., Sancho-Garnier H., Fender M. et al. (2000) Cervical cancer screening in France. *European Journal of Cancer* 36(17): 2215–2220.
5. Watt S. (2003) The cost of screening for breast and cervical cancer in France. *Bulletin Cancer* 90(11): 997–1004.
6. Schenck U. and Karsa L. (2000) Cervical cancer screening in Germany. *European Journal of Cancer* 36(17): 2221–2226.
7. American Cancer Society (2004) Cancer prevention and early Detection Facts and Figures.
8. DoH NHS cancer plan: A plan for investment, a plan for reform, 2000.
9. DoH Breast screening programme, England 2003–4. London, 2005.
10. Effect of NHS Breast Cancer Screening Programme on Mortality from Breast Cancer in England and Wales (2000) 1990–1998: comparison of observed with predicted mortality. *British Medical Journal*: 665–669.
11. Australian Government Department of Health and Ageing web site: www.breastscreen.info.au.
12. Australia's National Cancer Prevention Policy 06/2004.
13. Cancer Series, Number 25, The Australian Institute of Health and Welfare and the Australian Government Department of Health and Ageing for the BreastScreen Australia Program, Australian Institute of Health and Welfare, Canberra, 2003.
14. Australian Government Department of Health and Ageing web site: www.breastscreen.info.au.
15. DoH Serving Women for 15 years. NHS breast Screening programme Annual review (2003) DoH.

16. Ernst M. et al. (2004) Breast carcinoma diagnosis, treatment and prognosis before and after the introduction of mass mammographic screening. *Cancer* 100(7): 1337–1344.

17. Joensuu H. et al. (2004) Risk for distant recurrence of breast cancer detected by mammography Screening or other methods. *JAMA* 292: 1064–1073.

18. United States Preventive Services Task Force Report, Washington, 2004.

19. WHO World Cancer Report. IARC, Lyon, 2003.

20. UK CRC Screening Pilot Evaluation team (2003) Evaluation of the UK Colo-rectal cancer Screening Pilot.

21. Ramsey S.D. et al. (2003) Cancer-attributable costs of diagnosis and care for persons with screen-detected versus symptom-detected colo-rectal cancer. *Gastro-enterology* 125(6): 1645–1650.

22. Boncz I. et al. (2004) Health economics analysis of colo-rectal screening. *Hungarian Oncology* 48: 111.

23. Schwartz L. et al. (2004) Enthusiasm for cancer screening in the United States. *JAMA* 291: 71–78.

24. Gyrd-Hansen D., Holund B. and Andersen P. (1995) A cost-effectiveness analysis of cervical cancer screening: health policy implications. *Health Policy* 34: 35–51.

25. Sankaranarayanan R. et al. (2001) Effective screening programmes for cervical cancer in low- and middle-income developing countries. *Bulletin of the World health organization* 79: 954–962.

26. National Auditoffice (2004) Tackling cancer in England: saving more lives. NAO London.

4

Diagnostics

Introduction

We now come to the linked stages from diagnosis to treatment and care programmes. The new model increases the pressure for change and re-engineering across these areas of diagnostics, surgery, radiotherapy, and chemotherapy. In each area there are new conflicts:

- between new therapeutic options and available funding;
- between established professional hierarchies and new opportunities for teamwork;
- between traditional patient records and the quality of information technology required for managing personal care programmes;
- diagnosis, imaging, and the beginnings of personalised medicine.

Here we set out the technological agenda and ask, what developments are likely in diagnosis? Diagnosis is the identification of malignancy in patients but it also has a broader dimension including the issue of screening and predisposition to cancer considered in Chapter 3. Classically, diagnosis is a sequence of activities. It originates with research, with identifying the features that distinguish a normal cell from a cancer cell. Traditionally this has been a morphological analysis, using light microscopy. More recently there have been various dyes, stains, and special techniques developed and we now have sophisticated molecular reagents, based on antibodies that can discriminate with precision between a normal and a malignant cell. This research has to develop further as we need an evidence base to provide proof of concept that these tools are actually robust in terms of their ability to discriminate.

Transmitting information on new diagnostic techniques

If there is a general acceptance that there is a need for something that adds to the available tools (and this is one of the many things that needs to be determined rather carefully, since there are quite good tools for diagnosis already), what does that something add? And that of course includes some of the other dimensions such as cost and availability. Most cancer diagnosis is made by hospital doctors and pathologists and many of them do not attend specialist research meetings nor read specialist scientific journals. So there has to be a transmission of information amongst that community so that new tests can be introduced more widely. This is usually done using some sort of pilot system. Traditionally, it has not been well organised in that there are some enthusiasts in one or two institutions who have either been involved in developing or identifying a test and they push it forward, partly through their own enthusiasm and then this ripples out into the rest of the community. There has been little analysis of the economic impact of a diagnostic in the past.

Over the last 20 years the improving classification of disease is one of the specific breakthroughs in medicine. Therefore, when a new protein is discovered or a new molecular change is identified that is relevant to a particular disease we can introduce it into the clinic. There are now a plethora of additional tests to assist clinicians in establishing diagnosis and also to classify disease. The focus is a beginning to move away from diagnosis towards therapy planning and identifying what is the relevant treatment for an individual patient.

Currently the classification of most cancers is based on traditional morphological assessment and by looking at the biology of the disease and its long-term effects. It is not based on therapeutic intervention. Lymphoma classification, for example, over the last 20 years has moved from a morphological basis (an understanding of the cell types, shapes, and character through an evolution of understanding of what those cells are to a more informed morphological classification by understanding what those cells are doing and what proteins they contain). And the latest classifications for lymphoma no longer focus on any one of these areas. They do not focus exclusively on molecular biology or genetics although both play an important part, but look at a holistic approach in the clinical setting. That is the appropriate future paradigm for classification of all cancers as the potential therapeutic options increase.

What other things do we need to know about the tumour? If the patient has very early disease, surgical ablation is the most effective form of treatment, if there is no spread and it can be cured by simple removal. At the moment, staging is carried out in a very conventional way by the pathological examination of the tissues where we recognise that the tumour has a probability of spreading, for example, the lymph nodes in the axilla in a woman with breast cancer. These can be examined down the microscope to see if metastases have occurred. It may be that more effective imaging techniques will actually improve our ability to assess those non-operatively so the nodes will not need excision. This will reduce the distinct morbidity associated with these types of staging procedures. If we can improve imaging, then perhaps serum testing can actually become more effective rather than tissue diagnosis. Most new tests that come in, so long as they are cheap, are effectively evaluated by existing pathology laboratories so pathologists are seeking new knowledge all the time. As a leading breast pathologist states:

Clinicians are coming in all the time and saying can't we do this so every lab is very used to evaluating something in comparison to the existing profile. The problems come because tests are expensive they can't be resourced. There's a huge amount of evaluation going on routinely behind the scenes. Because most of these breakthroughs are actually very cheap, so we can actually run them. But if a reagent is extremely expensive or requires a new technology then there will be real concern about how to introduce it. The delays on expensive tests are huge at the moment. It takes years to get a development through the National Health Service. If it's in pathology and somebody comes out of the woodwork and says no, there's a problem here, then it's going to take you four to five years just to go through the green light procedures that are required. Then NICE comes in and you're not certain what they're going to say about it either. So there are huge delays in introducing expensive technologies. I don't think there's a delay in introducing cheap technologies in the NHS. They are very effective at introducing this as nobody notices or indeed cares.[1]

Training future pathologists and laboratory support staff is a major issue. There is a severe shortage of trained staff in the UK. There are 900 consultants and 300 vacancies at the moment so we are struggling to deliver just basic services, let alone move forward. There are two reasons for this situation. One is a manpower planning error that resulted in the training programme being stopped because there was a view that there were too many pathologists. We now have a hiatus with few pathologists coming out of training programmes to fill the vacancies. And the demand is expanding for all sorts

> **Box 4.1: Diagnosing cancer**
> 1. New diagnostic tests are introduced by enthusiasts and enter routine practice.
> 2. Specific diagnostics will accompany new therapies.
> 3. Pathologists will move away from morphological diagnostics into molecular assays.
> 4. There will remain a global shortage of pathologists.
> 5. Imaging and pathology will merge into a single discipline.
> 6. Computer-based decision support systems will enhance clinical judgement.
> 7. Future patients will interact with such systems from home.

of reasons; new technologies, litigation, and issues around patient management, the complexity of disease, and drug development using biomarkers, and surrogates. Pathologist reports in the last 10 years have quadrupled in length, which is a reflection of the information the pathologist is able to provide that is relevant to clinical care, so they are working harder in providing more information but there are fewer of them. (See Box 4.1.)

Imaging

Imaging has a lot to do with context. It is the picture that represents our understanding of whatever it is that is going on, be it in an art gallery or in a particular patient. We are shifting from the view of cancer as a disease of lumps and bumps to a disease of process. It has transformed from an anatomical disease to an abnormal molecular process. We are no longer talking about a disease that has to be removed but rather a disease more like diabetes that has to be identified at a certain point and regulated in subtle ways over a long period of time. Cancer is a regulatory problem rather than something that necessarily has to be eradicated.

Physicians use imaging in the management of most disease but in oncology we are trying to get a picture of what we are going to cut out, eradicate, define, or treat in some manner. Suddenly the paradigm we are imaging has shifted from the anatomic definition to identifying a process that is made more complicated by the observation that there is no single process that is absolutely unique to malignant disease.

There are four key questions:
1. What are we going to image?
2. Why are we going to image it?

3. What information are we going to take from of this process?

4. When and how often are we going to image to aid management decisions? Not only is the cultural context of our understanding of cancer changing, the cultural context of cancer around the world in the USA, Japan, France, Finland, and the UK is very different. In some respects, it is evidenced by a very interesting statistic on how much imaging is done in different countries. Looking at magnetic resonance imaging (MRI) as an example, in the USA there are 49 MRI machines per million of the population, in Japan 23, in France 8.2, in Finland 6.7, and in the UK 5.4. But if you look at overall cancer survival, we do not see a tenfold difference in our success at treating the disease.

Future predictions for imaging

What is going to be the function of imaging over the next 25 years? Imaging is a massive subject spanning the whole of science. Basically, we perturb a physical system and try to get a signal out of it. You can apply this to a single atom or the whole cosmos. Imaging will impact on all aspects of cancer care because it can non-invasively probe the molecular events as well as look at the greater picture of the events that define cancer *in vivo*. What is new is that we have always been used to conventional medical imaging giving us anatomical information. Now, we are beginning to image function and so everything is going to change.

Where will imaging impact be most? It will impact on clinical practice, on cancer drug development, on the relationship between animal and human experimentation, and ultimately on the creation of personalised cancer treatment programmes. From a clinical practice point of view, many of the morphological studies that we still do and the newer functional molecular studies will have an evidence based for their efficacy. We will determine objectively the right time to do a computed tomography (CT) scan to see whether a tumour has changed or not as opposed to being dictated by a specific protocol. We will have to demonstrate the cost benefit and cost effectiveness of new investigations. We will also have to validate our imaging against the underlying biological processes because if we are purporting to say that looking at the general physiology or a specific molecular target in a tissue, we need to validate this. We need to understand the relationship between the natural history of disease and specific molecular events. So what we will end up with is a situation whereby we could get a global view of the cancer process. Perhaps radiology and pathology will become the same thing in 25 years time because we will construct a map of abnormal vascularity, of pockets of hypoxia, of patches of abnormally proliferating tissue. Rather than looking at it on a 10-micrometer slice from a selective biopsy, we will be able to image the abnormal process in 3D across many centimetres without needing to insert any painful needles.

There is little difference in the requirements from imaging in the development of new anti-cancer drugs to routine clinical care it is just the emphasis. Sophisticated imaging, when properly validated, can provide vital information with key decision points in phases I, II, and III clinical trials. There are four points in which imaging will really impact in cancer by measuring angiogenesis, hypoxia, cell cycle modulation, and gene expression actually in patients. We are already a cross-disciplinary field. There is interaction between the physicists and oncologists. But we need to get to this new vision of actually looking at how the functional aspect of tumours is making new contacts with different scientific groups. The two that we have not yet engaged are chemists and biologists. To develop molecular targeted agents we need their skills. Our prediction is that there will be considerable impact of new technology from both optical imaging and hyperpolarised studies in magnetic resonance. The computer synthesis of artificially reconstructed images will help our understanding of the complex relationship between anatomy and disease process.

Funding new technology

How are we going to achieve all this? There is no doubt that imaging will remain a high cost resource so there are issues around how we are going to pay for all this wonderful new technology. Other than the conventional ways that we can think of funding these various developments, what we now want is a way forward in industry–academic collaboration, some of these based around private, dedicated phase I units. Imaging will have to start implementing guidance from regulatory bodies such as the Food and Drug Administration (FDA) and Evolution of Medicinal Products (EMEA). This should shorten the development process, in fact perhaps even halving it. Just as in pathology, there are nowhere near enough radiologists in this country.

How we are going to train them in a completely new discipline is a major issue. But in 25 years' time, we will not have radiology in the way we see it now. We will have disease specific imaging specialists. Let us also assume that in 2025 we have powerful functional imaging in its broadest sense. It already exists as a technology. We must assume that if we have a targeted therapeutic agent against a specific molecular defect it is very likely that we will also have some sort of targeted imaging agent.

The least controversial aspect about the new imaging technology is that it is going to lead to better selection of patients for local treatment modalities. It would be excellent if in 2025 we will no longer need surgeons and radiotherapists because everything is going to be revolving around drugs. We might still need surgeons and radiotherapists, possibly even more of them, because the way that they will be using their modality will be more sophisticated. So the issue of selecting patients, the issue of improved planning for surgery, and radiotherapy will consume far more skilled time and resources.

With functional imaging also comes the very real prospect that the imaging itself is going to be more sensitive. We will pick up smaller amounts of tumour than we currently can and inevitably this will link back to screening. However, there is a problem here in that a screening test has got to be something cheap, robust, and widely applicable and reliable. It may be some sort of functional imaging with a complex biologically targeted imaging agent. That may not be cheap but it could be very effective. Such tests may therefore be restricted to high-risk groups or to those able and willing to pay for them. This pattern is already emerging in the use of positron emission tomography (PET) to evaluate potential metastatic deposits.

Functional imaging

How do we select the treatment based on imaging? Will we just send the patient off for a conventional magnetic resonance scan and write up a request form for functional imaging say of HER-2neu expression? It is not going to be quite so simple because that is just one parameter and there are going to be whole molecular profiles that need to be built up. So functional imaging, particularly with the future ease with which we may be able to make probes, is not going to be quite as straightforward as conventional imaging, it could be very resource hungry.

The other factors we need to understand are the general features of a tumour such as vascularity, cell cycle, apoptosis, and differentiation. We are going to have to build up a composite picture to give us a reliable idea of what we are dealing with before we select the appropriate treatment. Another dimension to functional imaging is looking at heterogeneity. Spatial heterogeneity, where bits of the tumour really do look like the bit that the pathologist has taken and are there other bits of that tumour that are significantly different is clearly important. Certain features could be the determinants of the success or failure of treatment. The other aspect of heterogeneity is temporal. It may be that in response to treatments, particularly in response to newer biological agents, the tumour will change its characteristics. Imaging may detect the early signs that a tumour, which we are hitting in a very clever way, is starting to develop resistance quite early on. So not only is functional imaging going to be a more resource intensive as a one-off, it is also going to be something we cannot just do once and go away having given the patient their care plan. We are probably going to have to repeat the imaging process during the course of treatment and in follow up.

If we have targeting agents which can pick up just small amounts of disease, we may be going against the current trend of getting patients out of the hospital setting once they have had their radical treatment and back to the General Practitioners (GPs). If we develop effective functional imaging which can pick up small amounts of recurrent tumour and possibly treatments that can do something about it, that may be going to start pulling patients back into the hospital system. Finally, we need to consider the resource implications of imaging. This is going to be a very costly area to implement, both in terms of hardware, computer time, and staff. We have a real problem here because there is the great danger that this technology will only be accessed by the rich but not the poor, both globally and locally. Sophisticated imaging will have enormous costs and be developed by for-profit organisations that may well overplay its benefits at any point of time through skilled marketing direct to the end user – the patient.

Human eye versus computer recognition systems

Implicit in all current discussion on imaging is the production of pictures for humans to look at. But to what extent will machines be able to do this job in the future 2025 possibly rather better than human viewers? The human pattern recognition system was clearly a long way ahead of what machines can do and computer pathology recognition systems have been relatively slow in developing. On the other hand, US radiologists have been demonstrated to miss 30% of early breast cancers in routine mammography so the gold standard is not quite as shiny as we would hope. Do you really think by 2025 we are really going to be dependent on human reading of all of these images or is the whole process going to be much more automated? With functional imaging, it is already happening now because we can feed numerical data straight into a computer that can model using a pharmacokinetic programme in density perfusion studies. We do not need a trained morphological radiologist to interpret the data because the model just identifies that part of the tumour that is more permeable than other parts. Radiology will be very different and may merge with pathology giving a holistic approach to maximising information of clinical utility.

Improved diagnostics will increase prevalence

Over 3 million people in the UK will be living with cancer in 2025 mainly due to increasing prevalence. It will be true that many more old people will be living with one form of cancer or another as understood in 2005, but many more millions will be living with a predisposition for cancer and pre-cancer, as their genetic profile dictates, 3 million is therefore an underestimation. The drive to this change in the understanding of the nature of cancer will come from the increasing sophistication of old technologies, and the impact of this on the detection and diagnosis of cancer. This has huge implications for cancer treatment.

In 2005, most diagnoses of cancer depend on human interpretation of changes in cell structures seen down a microscope. By 2025, microscopes will be superseded by the new generation of scanners to perform the traditional role of microscopes, with the added advantage that they will detect molecular changes in living cells. These scanners will also build up a picture of cellular changes over time (they will "film" cellular activity rather than just take a photograph of a cell at one instance) as represented by the traditional biopsy. We will have the ability to probe molecular events that are markers for high cellular activity and, therefore, early malignant change.

This dynamic imaging will lead to more sensitive screening and treatments imaging agents which accumulate in cells exhibiting tell-tale signs of pre-cancer activity and will be used to introduce treatment agents directly, targeting the abnormal areas. Under certain circumstances detection and treatment could be simultaneous events as treatment will take place at a molecular level.

Imaging and diagnosis will be minimally invasive and enable the selection of the best and most effective targeted treatment. Even better imaging will be able to pick up pre-disease phases and deal with them at a stage long before they are currently detectable. These techniques will also be crucial in successful follow-up. A patient who has a predisposition to a certain cancer process will be monitored regularly and treatment offered when necessary. Not all cancers will be diagnosed in these earliest of stages – some patients will inevitably fall through the screening net. Nevertheless, there will be opportunities to offer them less invasive treatment than at present. Some therapeutic agents will be implanted into tumours obviating the need for surgical removal, other techniques will be much more developed such as radio-frequency ablation leading to such precision that only cancer tissue will be damaged.

Will traditional treatments such as surgery and radiotherapy continue to play their part? Yes, but in a vastly modified form, mainly as a result of the developments in imaging. Most significantly, surgery will become part of the integrated cancer care. Removal of tumours or even whole organs will remain necessary on occasions. However, the surgeon will be supported by 3D imaging, by radio-labelling techniques to guide incisions, and by robotic instruments. And although many of the new treatments made possible by improved imaging will be biologically driven, there will still be a role for radiotherapy (the most potent deoxy ribonucleic acid (DNA) damaging agent) to treat cancer with great geographical accuracy. The targeting of radiotherapy will be greatly enhanced by improvements in imaging enabling treatment to be more precise.

Combination therapy

Even in 2005, many cancer treatments were most effective given in combination with others. This will be just as true in 2025, but the focus of the combination will be different. Most treatment will be able to be performed on an outpatient basis, and the role of the clinician will be different to today. Changes in imaging and treatment delivery will mean that today's pathologists and radiologists will need similar skills. Only a few individuals may require formal medical qualifications and many treatments could be provided by technicians working to computer-aided protocols, and surgeons will find their roles changing as imaging and robotics take over many of their traditional tasks.

In addition to the reconfiguration and merging of the skills of clinicians, the delivery of care will also change. Minimally invasive treatments will reduce the need for long stays in hospital. As more patients are diagnosed with cancer, the need to provide the care close to where patients live will be both desirable and possible, and as this report will show later, expected. The prospect of highly sophisticated scanning equipment and mobile surgical units being transported to where they are required is not unrealistic. Technicians, surgical assistants, and nurses would provide the hands-on care, whilst technical support will be provided by the new breed of clinician, a disease-specific imaging specialist working from a remote site. Cost control will be an essential component of the diagnostic phase. Healthcare payers will create sophisticated systems to evaluate the economic benefits of new imaging and tissue analysis technology.

The new economic challenges of imaging and diagnostics

The main sources of additional workload can be listed as follows:

1. There will be increased requirements for diagnostics and imaging within established screening programmes. The breast-screening programme currently generates a significant demand for laboratory tests with about 100,000 people a year being sent for further test. Within this established screening programme clinical governance standards are likely to increase demand for the use of MRI scans (MRI scanning is more accurate than mammography in detecting cancer. However it did not reduce the need for breast biopsies[2]).
2. New screening programmes for colo-rectal and prostate cancer will generate increased demand.
3. New concerns about early diagnosis are likely to raise urgent referral as there will be greater concern amongst patients themselves.

4. New, more sophisticated treatment programmes will raise the requirement for laboratory diagnostics. Thus effective use of herceptin depends on the hercep b test. Within the UK this has already proved to be a bottleneck, limiting the use of the new therapy.
5. Increasing prevalence and risk management against recurrence.

The economic constraints

Along with increased demand is likely to come new economic constraints. Training future pathologists and laboratory support staff is a major issue. There is a severe shortage of trained staff in the UK. There are two reasons for this situation. One is a manpower planning error that resulted in the training programme being stopped because there was a view that there were too many pathologists. We now have a hiatus with few pathologists coming out of training programmes to fill the vacancies. And the demand is expanding for all sorts of reasons – new technologies, litigation, issues around patient management, the complexity of disease, and drug development using biomarkers and surrogates. Pathologist reports in the last 10 years have quadrupled in length – a reflection of the information the pathologist is able to provide that is relevant to clinical care. So they are working harder in providing more information but there are fewer of them.

The same situation is likely to affect many countries. In developed countries there may be some shift of the problem to middle income countries as countries seek to recruit abroad but this is unlikely to make much difference outside of capital cities. The likely reality is that cancer related workload in most laboratories will at least double over the next 10 years and that quality standards will become far stricter. The increase that has already taken place in the numbers of colonoscopies is significant. For the UK the numbers of classified diagnostic endoscopic examination of the colon using sigmoidoscopes rose from 77,322 in 1988/89 to 193,815 in 2002/3. This increase had taken place before the full impact of workload pressures and before the start of a formal screening programme.

There are no easy solutions to be found through increased automation as pathologists' judgement will remain vital. The international evidence, though circumstantial, is positive on the effectiveness of diagnostics and imaging. A recent Organisation for Economic Co-operation and Development (OECD)

Box 4.2: The new diagnostics

1. Radiology and pathology will merge into cancer imaging.
2. Dynamic imaging will create a changing image of biochemical abnormalities.
3. Imaging of hypoxia, vascularity, apoptosis, and specific gene expression will be possible.
4. Cancer changes will be detected prior to disease spread from primary site.
5. Greater precision in surgery and radiotherapy will be used for pre-cancer.
6. Molecular signatures will determine treatment choice.
7. Functional imaging will be routinely used to monitor response to therapy.
8. Cost control will be essential for healthcare payers to avoid inefficient diagnostics.

---

study showed that the US, Sweden, and Japan had some of the highest levels of MRI scanners per million population with 7.6 in the US and 8.0 in Sweden, while the UK and Canada (both of which have serious waiting time problems in cancer treatment) had some of the lowest. Thus the high level of equipment may well help the improved outcomes found in the US and Sweden by speeding up the treatment process. However, such advantages may be difficult to achieve in a future with faster increases in the diagnostic/imaging workload. The outlook for diagnostics and imaging increases the case for seeking new solutions for re-engineering the cancer treatment process (Box 4.2).[3]

REFERENCES

1. National Audit Office (2004) Tackling Cancer saving Lives. National Audit Office, London.
2. Bluemke D. et al. (2004) Magnetic resonance imaging of the breast prior to biopsy. *Journal of American Medical Association* 292: 2735–2742.
3. Organisation for Economic Co-operation and Development (2004). A Disease-based comparison of Health Systems. OECD.

5

Surgery

Surgery faces a huge challenge. Ninety per cent of all cancer patients who are cured completely are cured by surgery. Therefore, surgeons are often aggrieved when the entire cancer agenda seems to focus excessively on chemotherapy, radiotherapy, imaging and diagnostics: yet, "surgery remains the primary option for the cure of many cancers."[1] Surgery has become less invasive and yet remains a vital resource. Table 5.1 illustrates how overall survival and mortality following surgery has improved over recent decades.

With more day treatment and fewer major procedures the share of spending on surgery in total cancer spending has reduced. The main driver here has been the reduced number of in-patient days and lower complication rates. For the future, we anticipate important choices in terms of therapeutic options.

Principle drivers in developing surgery

There have been four main drivers of the surgical progress. The first has been the technology and devices industry. The second is the desire on the surgical community's part to excel. The third is patient and public expectations from surgeons. And, the last is progress in parallel fields of medicine. Fifty years ago, the factors that really prevented cancer surgery from taking off were pain, haemorrhage and sepsis and these are all now dealt with effectively as a result of progress in other fields of medicine, with surgery as the beneficiary.

The necessity for radical cancer operations has been a widely disputed issue for many years. Thirty years ago, there were still many radical mastectomies but now there are only very few. At the other end of the spectrum surgery has become far more radical in dealing with malignant liver disease for example. Primary hepatoma and liver metastases from bowel cancer can now be removed by aggressive surgery. Some patients with hepatoma in cirrhosis will have liver transplantation. Surgery for other common cancers,

Table 5.1. Changing rates in resectability, mortality and survival following surgery (all cancers)

Period	Resectability (%)	Mortality (%)	Survival (%)
Before 1970	37	15	38
Before 1980	53	13	52
Before 1990	58	5	55

Source: WHO, 2003.[1]

such as colon, lung and pancreas has changed little. There were colectomies, pneumonectomies and Whipple's operations (to remove the pancreas) 50 years ago. There remains a similar frequency of operations, but peri-operative mortality and safety has improved. Improved anaesthesia, intensive care and post-operative nursing have all played a role and will continue to do so. Robotics is likely to be one area for development with computer assistance in the planning and execution of surgery. Outside the UK, some surgeons already use three-dimensional imaging systems which not only show them a reconstructed representation of the liver but exactly where the tumour is and how many millimetres it is away from the portal vein and the hepatic artery. The imaging system provides them with the exact information on detailed anatomy to guide their incisions.

Techniques leading to less invasive surgery

Surgery is likely to become less invasive with smaller incisions using laparoscopic techniques. This leads to a shorter hospital stay for the patient and a lesser disturbance to their lives after the operation. As a consequence of all these advances, more radical and bigger operations will become possible. There will be varying developments by specialties with minimally invasive operations on the one hand and invasive mega-operations on the other. There will be more emphasis on intra-operative diagnosis. Ultrasound probing, radio-labelled imaging and even magnetic resonance imaging (MRI) guided surgery are all now available. There will be different diagnostic stains to identify malignancy. There might be fluorescent genes incorporated into cancers so that they will glow when the theatre lights are switched off and the tumour will glow.

There will be less use of blood and blood products: with moves beyond cell savers, which are already available to the use of artificial blood. Surgery will become more feasible in patients who are very ill. There will be intra-operative combinations of different treatment modalities, so a surgeon might resect a tumour and then at the same time ablate: irradiate that field with a portable tool in theatre. This has been already tried in pancreatic and breast cancer. Similarly, surgeons will give chemotherapy into a particular artery or vein with the hope of hitting any spreading cancer cells.

There will be newer adjunctive treatments, which will make radical surgery possible even for large tumours. Tumours previously labelled as unresectable are now being down staged by pre-operative chemotherapy. They are then resected and more chemotherapy follows on after that. Surgeons are already stretching the boundaries of resectable disease and will continue to do so. There are physiological manipulations now possible which might make certain operations feasible. There are more and more physiological manipulations which surgeons and radiologists are coming up with to make complex surgery possible.

Prophylactic surgery

One dilemma that will increasingly concern surgeons is pre-emptive surgery or prophylactic surgery. As screening tests become more and more accepted and widely used, there will be people identified as having a very high risk of a certain cancer. Inevitably the question will arise: why do we not take out the organ and eliminate the risk? Society will want this kind of prophylactic surgery to have a zero mortality as, after all, the patient appears well. We see the beginnings of this in colectomy for familial colo-rectal polyposis and in bilateral mastectomy and oophorectomy for women with certain genetic abnormalities.

In 25 years, surgery is still likely to remain a principal instrument of cure for cancers. The organ-specific approach to surgery will persist. Surgical oncology is on a possible route for development, yet in spite of support from World Health Organisation (WHO), we see this as unlikely. Surgery will remain organ based and this sub-specialisation will continue and become even more pronounced. Surgeons have already become, and will continue to evolve into, physicians who also operate.

Cancer as a chronic, controllable disease

Cancer will become like diabetes, treated with various biological therapies to keep the cancer under control. That prediction is correct for metastatic disease but it is extremely unlikely to apply to early localised disease without further spread. Surgery will remain the main modality for the treatment of this stage of disease. Undoubtedly the advances in molecular biology will lead to earlier detection, and therefore, we can predict that the number of prophylactic procedures will increase because we will be able to identify those at high risk early on.

Technological advances and the magnitude of surgery will profoundly influence the future of cancer surgery. Surgery for cancer in general will become less radical. Forty years ago, radical mastectomy was the standard of care for breast cancer. Now we have moved towards excision biopsy for most patients. In the future many cancer patients will be treated in the out-patient setting using radio frequency delivered by image guidance. There are three studies now showing that this technique can be successful in more than 90% of patients. The challenge for us is to predict the response to radio-frequency ablation by MRI. But the technology is showing great promise and small tumours in the future are likely to be treated in the out-patient setting.

In breast cancer, axillary node clearance has been standard practice for a very long time. Now surgeons are becoming less invasive in their approach. They are using the sentinel node biopsy, which very shortly will become the standard of care in patients with clinically negative axillary disease. This allows identification of the node that is most likely to drain the breast tumour and to dissect out only that node to gain all the information we need about the stage the cancer is at, and then treat the patient accordingly, rather than removing a large number of lymph nodes. So axillary surgery has become less invasive and that trend will continue.It is very possible in the future even that the sentinel node biopsy, which we regard now as a new technique, may not be necessary. More effective, less invasive imaging and biopsy will provide us with more information.

Computer-assisted surgery

One of the main features of the surgical future will be the increasing use of computer-assisted surgery with robotics playing an important role. There are encouraging results from randomised control trials in Europe, demonstrating that laparoscopic colectomy has equivalent recurrence or disease-free survival to that of open colectomy, and the earlier concerns about metastases at the site of the port of the laparoscopic equipment seem to be fading. So, we predict in the future that colo-rectal surgery or colo-rectal resection would be performed endoscopically, probably with computer-assisted surgery. Again, rather than dissecting the whole of the mesorectum or mesocolon, which contains the lymph nodes, a form of sentinel node biopsy is likely to be developed.

Computer-assisted surgery has many advantages; it is minimally invasive, more precise, and it facilitates surgery and access. For example, an organ like the prostate is very difficult to access surgically; the dissection involved is fraught with complications. The other feature of computer-assisted surgery is the navigational component that gives us more precise information on the state of the disease and the anatomy of the organ concerned. The benefits are already being demonstrated in various studies. There is evidence that computer-assisted surgery is associated with less pain, bleeding and shorter hospitalisation.

Surgery in 2025

Let us try to predict what the operating room would look like in 2025. We expect that this will be large as there will be an increased number of robotic arms involved. There will be a computer and a surgeon sitting behind it directing the robotic arms to perform the actual procedure. However, controlling this procedure does not really need to be performed in the same operating room. There are already examples of laparoscopic colectomies performed in Europe by a surgeon sitting in the USA. So the combination of the navigational and robotics will need to be linked together to guide the surgery, and therefore, we expect that there will be a telesurgical workstation in the operating room. Obviously, these advances will have huge implications for hospital design.

The implications of these advances are important in planning health-care provision. Hospitalisation will be shortened, the conventional wards we are used to where a patient coming in for a colectomy will stay for probably 10 days is likely to disappear. There will be shorter stay wards, if not day surgery, for most procedures. This is crucial for planning developments in the hospital setting. There will be fewer and fewer in-patient beds. We have discussed the adaptations in the operating room where there will be high capital costs involved. To buy a robot like the Da Vinci surgical device, the most popular robot currently in the USA, costs about $1.5 million, so the capital cost is high. Nevertheless, that capital cost will be partly offset by the other benefits associated with the technology, namely the shorter hospitalisation and the lower morbidity. Therefore, there will be fewer specialised centres treating a larger number of patients and we need to consider the total financial implications. Insurance companies will need to think about the new reimbursement policies. Larger centres treating larger numbers of patients but at fewer places are inevitable. Patients will have to travel further. Several studies have shown that patients do not mind travelling for better treatment. Obviously, there are those who will have practical difficulties such as disability. Society has to provide the required transport for them, but in general, patients actually do not mind travelling longer distances for better care for cancer.

New training requirements

The nursing role will be shifted from the hospital to the community and that is something that needs to be taken into account by planners. We will begin seeing organ-specific specialties. For example, there will be a liver unit, where a liver physician, pathologists, biochemists and surgeons will work as one group. All these specialists will be linked through sophisticated IT equipment to facilitate transmission of information. There will also be a need to revise the medical and nursing curriculum, and it is very important to take training requirements into account. A steep learning curve is one of the problems that we are going to face. For example, for those who want to do laparoscopic colectomy – because laparoscopic colectomy is not currently the standard practice. But it is going to become the standard of care in the near future and unless we have taken that into account in designing our training programmes, we will have problems in having the necessary expertise available.

Predicting future costs of cancer surgery

There are very different views on future costs of cancer surgery. One prediction is that costs will increase yet another suggests costs should decrease
because of the lower length of hospital stay, minimally invasive procedures
and earlier detection. However, the costs per treatment will actually increase
because there will be much more effort put into a shorter period of time
compared with now so that the shorter length of time actually increases the cost
per patient day. Supply is more readily available and beds will be more accessible, and essentially, you get life in a system where there has traditionally
been a supply blockage. Costs will increase, not necessarily because of the
technology or the length of stay, but because access to the service will
become more available.

Sometimes we get increasingly worried about where the patient fits in all
this, the person with the spirit, soul and emotions. Surgeons take people to
the brink of death and bring them back again. For the average human being
that is a fairly daunting experience and if we have very short hospital stays,
with people coming in for a something-ectomy, with no idea how serious it is,
then what it is going to be like afterwards? What are the possible long- or
short-term side-effects? They may feel very lost, lonely and worried when
they go home. Close post-operative follow-up by telephone, email and video
linkage will be necessary. We cannot emphasise enough how important and
traumatic an event illness is in people's lives. Counselling and psychosocial
support will be vital and there will be a change in the way these are delivered.
Currently, a patient coming for a breast cancer operation is seen by the
breast care counsellor during hospitalisation; that role will be shifted to the
community in future.

Re-engineering surgery: summary

The first challenge will be in improving the information base both for better
communication with patients and for teamwork amongst clinicians and support staff:
1. As cancer becomes a longer-term illness patients will require more information about options for treatment and possible benefits and side-effects.
   With more information there has already been a change in perspectives

on surgery for prostate cancer. More patients are opting for radiotherapy and for England the number of Trans-Urethral Resection of the Prostrate (TURPS) operations has reduced from 80,000 in 1995 to 40,000 in 2003.

2. With more combined programmes including surgery/radiotherapy/chemotherapy, there will be greater need for multi-disciplinary teamwork. Surgery will get a new focus (and a wider recognition of its role) from this new kind of teamwork. There will also be new concerns with care programmes and protocols. The evidence base of cancer surgery will become more varied. Already in the UK, National Institute for Clinical Excellence (NICE) has advised against the use of laparoscopic surgery in colo-rectal cancer. The percentage of cases treated with these methods remained unchanged at 0.1% between 1998 and 2001.[2]

3. There will be new issues about concentrating treatment for rarer types of surgery in fewer centres. This is being done for surgery in prostate cancer in the UK, and there is strong evidence from the US that for specialised surgery in pancreatic and kidney cancer larger units get survival results that are 30–40% better than units that do few procedures. Such differences are not, however, found in colo-rectal cancer surgery where results in larger units are only 3–4% better.[3]

4. The surgical role will be more divided between relatively limited procedures or early cancers and more complex operations for older higher-risk patients, often with more advanced cancer. At this extreme, surgery will become more involved with "difficult-to-treat" patients. Thus, longer-term expenditure on surgery will rise even if the initial episode cost falls.

REFERENCES

1. WHO (2003) *World Cancer Report.* IARC, Lyon, France.
2. *NICE Guidance on the Use of Laparoscopic Surgery for Colorectal Cancer. Technology Appraisal 17.* 2000.
3. Begg C. et al. (1998) Impact of hospital volume on operative mortality for major cancer surgery. *JAMA* 280, 1747–1751.

6

Radiotherapy

Radiotherapy will experience increased demand as result of rising prevalence of prostate cancer in particular, along with other cancers, which are heavy users of this therapy, but it will also be affected by changes in techniques which require more intensive planning:

1. There will be a requirement for more primary treatment of prostate cancer. As a result of increased incidence and shifts in preference away from surgery towards radiotherapy there will be an increase in demand. As cancer becomes a longer-term illness there will also be an increased requirement for palliative radiotherapy and treatment on a prophylactic basis.

2. Brachytherapy will improve the patient experience by reducing serious side effects. This improvement in quality will also increase demand while at the same time raising cost and the requirement for technical skills.

Technical advances in radiotherapy

Over the last 20 years the indications for radiation therapy have doubled, yet there are still many experts who feel radiotherapy will soon be obsolete. However, just as for surgery, there is little justification for this future scenario. Technological advances have led to the ability to plan and deliver non-uniform distributions of radiotherapy dose: molecular imaging allows us to look at the function of tumours so we can map resistant areas and titrate treatment (we can now selectively avoid normal tissues of functional importance), radiotherapy is the only treatment which can be modulated in time and space. At the other end of the spectrum, as well as its curative role, radiation therapy is the most cost effective palliative treatment we have. If many cancers are to become chronic illnesses, its role will become increasingly important perhaps through open access services directly to patients. Similarly, the emergence of biologically targeted therapies will expand rather than contract the role of radiotherapy.

Radiotherapy: where is its place in the plethora of cancer treatments?

We must ask why radiotherapy is so undervalued. Perhaps, it is because it has been around for over 100 years, perhaps it relates to the emergence of long-term effects related to a period when we were unable to shape the treatment and spare normal tissues and we did not understand the importance of scheduling (in terms of total dose, dose per treatment and overall time), perhaps it is related to the expectation that soon the right combinations of drugs will cure cancer. Whatever the reason there is no doubt that such prejudice is the greatest challenge to radiation therapy. It is reflected in the under-investment in research and equipment and it is reflected in media stories: the words associated with chemotherapy ("breakthrough", "new", "cure") are different from those associated with radiotherapy ("only radiotherapy", "exhausting", "burning", "damage". In a 1999 survey, radiation therapists were significantly less likely to be described as "top cancer doctors" compared with medical oncologists or surgeons.

The challenge for radiotherapy

The greatest challenge for radiotherapy is to acknowledge the current prejudices, deal with them through education and invest in equipment, skilled staff, and research and development to fully realise the potential of this excellent therapy. In order to figure out where we are going to go in 25 years' time, we have to look at where we have come from to get a general feel of the direction of travel. What happens with 100 typical patients with cancer today? Around 20 of them will have relatively trivial conditions such as skin cancers and carcinoma *in situ* that can be ablated in a relatively straightforward way with quite simple treatments. Around 40 will have localised disease that can be cured either with surgery or radiotherapy. The best choice will vary from site to site in the body. So for colon cancer, it is undoubtedly surgery that is the principal curative modality whereas for lymphoma radiation therapy is better. For some diseases such as prostate and bladder cancer, both modalities can be used and many of these patients are cured. We then end up with 40 patients who have metastatic disease and who are not cured. They started off with advanced disease even though it may not have been detectable by staging investigations. Subdividing these further, because only about 5 of these 40 have a curable cancer – a lymphoma, leukaemia or testicular tumour. And only 2 of them are actually cured by chemotherapy and these are the 2, of course, that the medical oncologists get very excited about. But they are actually a very small component of the entire cancer problem. The other 35 will have incurable cancer – metastatic colo-rectal cancer, lung cancer, breast cancer, prostate cancer and so on. For these patients, the best we can hope to do is offer effective palliation as we have already heard, radiotherapy is a very effective way of doing this.

We can predict that as we get increased awareness of cancer and better diagnostic tests we will see a shift from advanced disease to the localised disease. Prostate cancer is a good example. Thirty years ago 80% of patients presented with metastatic prostate cancer. In the USA, this is now less than 5% reflected in an increased demand for locally targeted therapies, either surgery or radiotherapy. So in terms of where we are now and where we are likely to be going, it is likely to be towards more locally targeted therapies. There is going to be a much more prominent role for precision radiotherapy.

Advances in radiotherapy

The majority of advances in radiotherapy that we have had over the last century have been physics driven. X-rays were discovered by Röentgen at the end of the 19th century and used therapeutically for skin tumours within a year or so of their discovery. It gradually extended its usefulness as the technologies improved with higher energy, more penetrating beams – 250 kV orthovoltage, through cobalt and then to linear accelerators that allowed us to treat progressively more deep-seated tumours. This was coupled to advances in imaging and beam shaping so that doctors and health professionals could reduce morbidity by cutting out the corners of the fields and shaping them more precisely around the tumour and avoiding sensitive normal tissues. But the physics driven advances in radiation have largely run their course and the future, in terms of radiation therapy, is biological. There are possible, even likely, advances in the biological component of radiotherapy to maximise its power to destroy cancer cells selectively.

This can be illustrated with two examples: bladder cancer is a common cancer with 5000 deaths per year in the UK. We treat localised bladder cancer either with surgery or radiotherapy. If we take 100 patients with bladder cancer and give them radiotherapy, 60 will get durable local control in the bladder. They will not get further cancer back in their bladder. So they have an outpatient treatment that lasts between 4 and 6 weeks, they get a bit of diarrhoea, a bit of dysuria, but at the end of it they have still got a functioning bladder. Many studies show that their bladders will operate optimally for the rest of their lives. However, 40 of the 100 patients that receive radiotherapy will get a local recurrence. Those patients then go on to have a cystectomy as well. But the majority are better off than having a cystectomy up front. A surgeon reports on how national policies may have led to unexpected and counter-productive changes in choice of therapies:

There is a law of unintended consequences when we introduce a well-meaning policy. When the NICE guidance came out for urological cancer, there was a recommendation that in order to be a surgeon claiming specialisation in bladder cancer, at least five procedures a year should be performed. The intention being that if a surgeon performed fewer procedures patients should be referred into the centre in order to concentrate expertise. Now the minute the guidance was circulated, the radiotherapy demand for bladder cancer dropped by 75%. All surgeons doing up to four operations a year suddenly realised they had to do more or stop altogether. So they stopped referring the patients for radiotherapy. The consequence was that the wrong patients were getting surgery. They were not referring them into colleagues. The policy was well meaning but actually the consequences were serious. There is no evidence of a difference in outcome depending on which treatment is used but the consequence of this particular NICE guidance is that there are many people now walking around without bladders unnecessarily.[1]

Proteomic and deoxyribonucleic acid (DNA) chip type technology will allow the prediction of outcomes from different therapies. So if, for example, we are able to predict which of the 60% of the bladder cancer patients were going to get a good response to radiotherapy then we would offer them radiotherapy because they are going to keep their bladder. We may also be able to identify which ones are going to get severe late effects or bad acute reactions to their radiotherapy. So we can select the patients for whom radiotherapy is a good treatment and those for whom surgery might be a better option. One of the consequences of that is, that even without the efficacy of the treatment changing, the outcome of radiotherapy will get better because we can go from a 60% response rate to a 100% response rate if we have a perfect predictive constellation of tests.

Predictive testing

There are going to be big changes coming from this sort of predictive testing. This same sort of testing is also going to give us new targets, for example BCL-2 expression in bladder cancer. We know that over expression of this protein is an adverse prognostic factor leading to a worse outcome with radiotherapy and chemotherapy. We can envisage treatments that target the BCL-2 protein specifically in patients who over express it. In this way, a non-responder to radiotherapy or chemotherapy can be turned into a responder. There is going to be a large increase in novel treatments.

One of the features that is strikingly absent from the radiotherapy compared to the chemotherapy literature is response analysis. If we imagine that instead of calling it radiotherapy we call it a drug – photomycin. Medical oncologists would work out the maximum tolerated dose and then put it in combination. They would be combining it with other drugs using different schedules. But the radiotherapy literature is tunnel-vision and tends to be focused on giving ever bigger doses to ever more tightly defined volumes of tissue. But we know that most cancer treatments work best in combination. A very simple example of this is again prostate cancer. Radiotherapy given alone to patients with localised prostate cancer that is relatively advanced – T3/T4 tumours results in 55% of the patients being alive 5 years later. Forty five per cent of them will die: even though we have what appears to be an effective salvage therapy with androgen removal or blockade using luteinising hormone-releasing hormone (LHRH) agonists. But if we give an LHRH agonist at the same time as radiotherapy, 80% of the patients are alive 5 years later. So the patients have had the same treatment but they have had it together up front. There is a massive unmined dataset to explore to sort out the huge numbers of potential combinations. Over the next 20 years such a strategy could improve outcomes substantially.

Economic consequences of predictive testing

What are the economics consequences of predictive testing? The costs may actually come down because we are more likely to get the right treatment to the right patient. The consequences of failure are usually expensive so there may be a potential overall cost saving. On the other hand, there are clearly going to be cost increases if we are giving more complex treatments combined with chemotherapy, combined with small molecule inhibitors that target particular oncoproteins. So there is going to be a complex involvement of competing costs. I have a feeling that the overall effect is going to be an increase in cost but hopefully this will be matched by an improvement in outcomes.

Today, we essentially have external beam treatment, where we can change the shape of the fields very precisely and we have radioactive sources that we can put directly into tumours of the prostate or of the cervix. We can also administer radioactive substances, radioisotopes, which pass through the circulation or be instilled in body cavities. There is panoply of ways in which to deliver radiation: and currently in conventional radiotherapy we have simulators that can localise the cancer and separate machines that deliver the radiation. There is a whole array of imaging modalities which are now coming on stream and what we will see in 2025 is a constellation of these imaging facilities directly linked to our radiation delivery systems.

We can call these "Centres for Biological Imaging for Adaptive Radiotherapy" or CEBARS. There are already forerunners being built in North America as cooperative networks evaluate the implications of new technologies. We will have computer tomography (CT) scans, magnetic resonance imaging (MRI), MR spectroscopy and positron emission tomography (PET). But what is very exciting about PET scanning is that it gives us biological information that we can place within the anatomical framework of a CT or MRI scan. When we are using our planning systems that are CT based, we will be able to see where the cancer is in our treatment field and how it is responding. That is a quantum leap in terms of treatment facilities both for targeting the cancer and assessing response. There will be a lot of implications for this because from PET scanning we will have information about the biochemical framework of the tumour. With parallel computing we will be able to examine a large number of biological parameters, and see what those activities are within the tumour. We will then target the dose to those particular parts of the tumour: a sort of "radiotherapy online". We will follow the situation on a day-to-day basis from dynamic information that we are collecting from functional imaging. We will be targeting dose to different parts of the tumour and then we will be seeing how that correlates with local control. This is going to require very large computational groups to analyse the data and we will need to change the skill set of the radiotherapist.

Intensive modulated radiotherapy

We already have intensive modulated radiotherapy (IMRT). This is essentially a technique that allows us to shape the beam more accurately to the tumour and spare normal tissues. A course of traditional radiotherapy is given in a number of treatments over a period of 3–6 weeks. We then see what the response is. With PET we will be in a position to assess the response of the tumour almost instantaneously. There is already good data from head and neck cancer that we can detect response in PET before we see shrinkage of neck nodes. So rather than simply giving a whole course of radiotherapy and then seeing what happens, we will be in a position to do a PET scan after the first three fractions and see if there is a trend towards response. If there is not, we will move to another form of treatment. That, on the one hand, creates more imaging demand but at the same time, it means we will save patients from additional toxicity.

Tomotherapy

There are some other technological advances, such as tomotherapy being installed in the USA. This is essentially a system that uses a holistic delivery system for radiotherapy in which both the planning and delivery systems are integrated with the treatment couch movement. There is no separate simulator and treatment facility – they are integrated into one unit. The advantage is that the dose outside the volume of the tumour is lower and therefore there is more flexibility in the kind of treatment fields that can be delivered.

Ion therapy

There are exciting developments in ion therapy. This is a form of treatment that produces intense radiation within a very confined volume. There now six centres in mainland Europe that are evaluating this for traditionally radio-resistant tumours of small volume. These include basal chordomas inside the skull. So, we can see that there may be transnational facilities which will be treating a thousand patients a year and we will have to agree arrangements with these countries as to where these patients are going and how the centre will be reimbursed. There are implications in terms of access to care. If there is great capacity in other parts of Europe, we are going to have to come to agreement on national standards of waiting times.

Robotics

There will also be developments in robotics because there are elements of radiation delivery that really lend themselves to this. There is already a system developed in the USA called the cyberknife. This is essentially a linear accelerator linked to a CT scanner. The patient has their tumour imaged by the CT that pre-programs the robotic arm to deliver radiotherapy from a series of six angles on a sequential basis. It stops at a certain number of nodes on the way in the sequence of delivery to check that the imaging is correct and that the patient has not moved. Another area of potential advance is the positioning of radioactive substances directly into the tumour – interstitial therapy. Until now this has been carried out manually so it is a highly operator-dependant technique. The skill set for these ranges very widely across the UK and we probably ought to concentrate it into four dedicated centres. In prostate cancer for example, we place 10 or more radioactive needles into the gland. The more needles put in, the longer it takes and the greater the prostatic oedema. So if we have techniques that could actually place the needles directly into the prostate under robotic control, it could judge exactly the distance that they have to go in so reducing the time and number, and therefore minimising the swelling. This could apply to many different application types – needles, seeds, colloids and particles.

Boron neutron capture therapy

Another interesting development is boron neutron capture therapy (BNCT). This is based on rather ancient physics. A particular isotope of boron in the presence of a low energy neutron field captures the neutrons and releases alpha particles. Now this sounds very obscure but the significance of it is that we can boronate drugs that are actively taken up by tumours. We can use a low energy neutron beam to produce this reaction at a level below that of ionization so it is biologically a relatively inert beam. But where the neutrons encounter boron there is an intense release of radiation so giving biologically targeted radiation. It is an old idea and part of the reason that it has been difficult to get it to work is because a traditional neutron beam is hard to obtain. Treatments have been given by taking patients to nuclear reactors. A whole series of patients were treated in Japan in the 1980s and now linear accelerator based machines that will produce a neutron beam are available.

Nanotechnology

There is also the application of nanotechnology. Essentially, we have a disease at a molecular level and we need to get treatment devices that get in at that level. There are molecular tools in production which are sub-cellular in size and which can be controlled externally by acoustic signals, that can be targeted to particular parts of the tumour and used, for example, to measure the level of oxygen within a cancer. This level may relate to radio-resistance. There are systems under development that will deliver oxygen to particular parts of a tumour.

The scenario within the CEBAR would have patients who had molecular nanotechnology devices in place and we would be able to target the delivery of oxygen to those particular parts of the tumour that have a deficit and we would see how those changes correlate with local control.

So there is a whole sea change in terms of technological delivery. If surgery eradicated 90% of localised cancer but a third of those patients died of local failure then if we could increase local control to 100%, we would increase survival from 45% to 60%.

Economic constraints

There are important staffing implications: between now and 2025 we need to make sure that we have the physicists, dosimetrists and radiographers to deliver this treatment. Brachytherapy takes around 50% more time for physicists in treatment planning and around 20% more time from radiographers in actually delivering treatment. There is certainly scope for using less highly trained assistants to carry out a support role. One case study in the South of England showed the gains possible from this:

Around 10 years ago, we had one of the worst waiting lists in the country for radiotherapy. We were underprovided for at all sorts of levels and partly that is been addressed by

---

Box 6.1: Radiotherapy

1. Increased conformal radiotherapy will deliver greater precision.
2. Biological selectivity will be enhanced by personalised scheduling.
3. Novel technologies will deliver systemic radiotherapy.
4. Increased centralisation of sophisticated imaging and delivery systems.
5. More informed choice between surgery and radiotherapy.
6. Open access palliative treatment for patients with painful metastases.

---

new equipment but over the last 2 years, we have gone from having an eight week waiting list to no waiting list at all for radiotherapy, either radical or palliative. We have done this by adjusting the skill mix. So we have stripped out the unnecessary use of highly skilled radiographers to move patients in and out of machines by creating radiographer helpers often in the teeth of resistance from the radiographers who saw themselves as being encroached upon. But once we did it and they realised they were not running around after notes and X-rays anymore, they were a lot happier and we found our vacancy rate dropped, our staff retention went up. The more it went up the more the waiting times came down and the happier everybody was. The patients were happier, the staff got less abuse and we now have very good retention figures. So we can do a lot with skill mix adjustment in cancer care.

However, such change will not create all the additional time required both for additional demand and for changed methods. Joint programmes are required between users and companies to develop technologies that would assist in more rapid treatment with a greater element of automation. There are also likely to be requirements or more hub-and-spoke systems so as to improve patient access. Treatment planning would be concentrated on a few centres but there would be more local access for further courses. Radiotherapy in the past has become increasingly concentrated on a few centres by the complexity and cost of equipment. The care challenges for the next phase will include many more elderly patients who cannot travel long distances on a daily basis. The new systems have to deliver quality and to meet technical and safety requirements (Box 6.1).

REFERENCES

1. Personal Communication.

7

Chemotherapy

Generic chemotherapy drugs

Chemotherapy faces a period of great change. There are pressures to reduce the cost of drug purchase and administration for established drugs. Some indications of the pressure in the USA include new Medicare schedules for payment of oncologists, which reduce funding for administration of chemotherapy. The reduced funding for branded drugs will encourage the purchase of generic drugs and these now have greater professional acceptability than before. According to the former Director of the Food and Drug Administration (FDA) and present Director of Medicare Dr Mark McClellan:

> We just all need to spend our money better, to take steps like encouraging more widespread use of generic drugs where they are available and while there are effective therapy alternates.[1]

More standard therapies will be available in oral form, which will further reduce the administration costs of drugs. Such a change will have particular implication for the health system in Germany where chemotherapy has often been delivered on an in-patient basis. A new range of drugs will become available for later stage cancer. These biological acting drugs will cost $10,000–15,000 per treatment cycle and will be aimed either at rarer cancers or the later stages of more common cancers. The actual cost of the drug will be only one part of the total cost which will often involve additional time from specialists and diagnostic tests. These new therapies will raise challenges of targeting. Even US experts as the Chief Medical Officer have expressed some doubts about the affordability of these drugs for all patients, which point to the necessity for targeting. As the Chief Medical Officer of the American Cancer Society recently stated:

> The country cannot afford these expensive biologic drugs in the treatment of metastatic cancer in order to gain a few months survival. But the country can afford the use of these

drugs if they are used in conjunction with other chemotherapy agents to improve the cure rate in metastatic cancer.[2]

The new change also presents a challenge in service re-organisation since the cost of specialist centres are likely to rise both through concentration of treatment and through the increase in numbers of patients seeking treatment. Thus, the costs of early stage cancer treatment may well fall with more day treatment and the use of generic drugs, while the costs of later stage treatment will rise.

The therapeutic agenda

When we look back at the history of oncology we are humbled by the enormous power of some of the things we have been able to do. Patients with testicular cancer, Hodgkin's disease, and even breast and colon cancer patients for whom we can offer significant life-changing intervention with chemotherapy. We are also humbled by the limits of what we have been able to achieve and the frustrations we have experienced. There are a number of phrases that we have been exposed to over the years that reflect the kind of journey it has been; single agents, combined agents, schedule dependence, dose intensity, dose density, big dose, small dose, killing cells, regulating cells, and more recently, highly specific targeting and dirty specificity.

There are four key questions:
1. What is the biological model for giving chemotherapy?
2. What are our measures of success to be – the end points and the surrogates?
3. What are our therapeutic goals?
4. How does that model take into account our respect for the person and our community values?

How effective is chemotherapy?

Chemotherapy effectiveness can be divided into three groups of cancers. In the first we can achieve a high percentage of complete response and a high cure rate; a second where we have a high complete response rate but the cure rate is low and another group where chemotherapy is really not very beneficial. The problem with chemotherapy for advanced disease is that the good group contains less than 5% of all patients with cancer. If we look back at the last 25 years, the only disease that has shifted groups is testicular cancer. If there are

> **Dramatic increase in molecular therapies**
>
> • Sequencing and bioinformatics
> • Expression vectors for target production
> • Predictive ability of 3D structural biology
> • Robotic high throughput screening
> • Combinatorial chemistry
> • Platform approach to drug discovery
> • Huge increase in number of targets

Figure 7.1

going to be improvements, we would expect to see a shifting of disease from the poorer to the better groups: that would be the clearest signal of success.

There is currently much excitement about chemotherapy based on; the human genome programme, bioinformatics, robots for high throughput screening, *in silico* drug design, and whole platforms such as the kinases for which to create drugs. New biomarkers identifying pharmacodynamic (PD) end points will be discovered so we can actually measure if the drug is hitting on its target by just taking a sample of tissue from the patient. We now have surrogate end points and molecular signatures to predict response to different agents. The pathology of the future is not going to be about microscopic morphology, it will be about identifying for molecular patterns that rationally guide therapy (Figures 7.1 and 7.2).

Clinical trials for new chemotherapies

There are currently over 500 drugs in clinical trial for cancer of which about 300 are against specific molecular targets. By 2006, competitive intelligence suggests there will be 2000 compounds and probably by 2010 it will be 5000 compounds. There are patterns evolving as the industry has very little imagination. At the moment the main theme is small molecules. Monoclonal antibodies, cancer vaccines, and gene therapy are on trial in a smaller scale but the emphasis is on small molecules. There are only seven biological processes we need to consider:

1. Cell cycle
2. Apoptosis

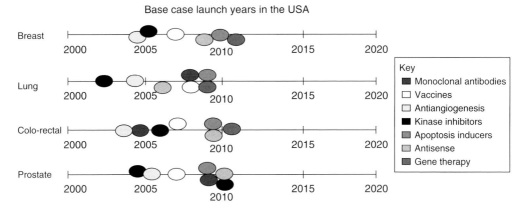

Figure 7.2
Source: Bosanquet and Sikora, 2004.[3]

3. Signal transduction
4. Angiogenesis
5. Inflammation
6. Invasion
7. Differentiation.

Nearly 90% of the entire global portfolio of cancer drugs in development revolves around small molecules targeting the controls of these processes. The other approach is random screening of agents from natural sources. Taxol from the yew tree, Vincristine from the periwinkle and Doxorubicin from a lichen. The drugs we have got now come from natural sources and there are still huge programmes to look for more. We do not know where they are going to come from and it is very difficult to design a logical process. Rational drug design and random screening are the two hunting grounds for the future. McKinsey estimates that at the moment the cost of cancer drugs is $21 billion globally, of which about $14 billion is spent in the USA and $7 billion in the rest of the world. McKinsey's forecast is for an expansion to $65 billion and increased numbers of cancer patients in an ageing population, increased patient advocacy, and new agents. And if we assume we get effective drugs into the clinic and it all pans out as planned, then by 2025, the cancer drug market will be worth $300 billion globally (Figures 7.3 and 7.4).[4]

Cancer drug sales – actual

Cancer drug sales: 2003
Total $22 billion

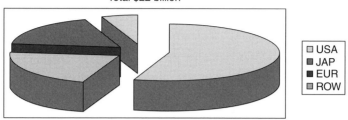

- USA
- JAP
- EUR
- ROW

Figure 7.3

Cancer drug sales – projected

Cancer drug market set to quadruple by 2015

Global cancer market by sector

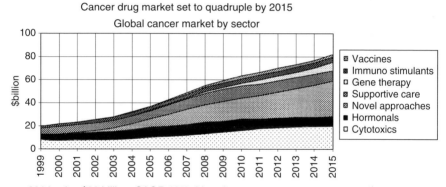

- Vaccines
- Immuno stimulants
- Gene therapy
- Supportive care
- Novel approaches
- Hormonals
- Cytotoxics

- 2014 sales $80 billion, CAGR 12% driven by:
  - New technology, particularly biologically targeted therapies
  - Earlier intervention
  - Patient number (ageing population, other diseases controlled)

Figure 7.4

The effective use of diagnostics will become a central component for optimal cancer patient management. Diagnostics can be divided into clinical imaging and sample analysis in the laboratory. The latter can be split into assays for specific molecules and more holistic measurements of ribonucleic acid (RNA), protein or modified structures. Increasingly, drug developers are turning to sophisticated diagnostic technologies to guide patient selection for trials of novel agents. Diagnostic tools such as biomarkers, surrogates, functional imaging, and molecular signatures are becoming essential in guiding critical decisions in the development of novel anti-cancer agents.

Translational research

Imaginative clinical assays, often using repeat biopsies of tumour and normal tissue, pose significant technical, logistical and ethical challenges. This area of research will drive much closer interactions between discovery and clinical groups, the creation of imaginative partnerships between academic centres and industry, and the formation of specialist, diagnostic contract research organisations (CROs). Multinational, consolidated pharmaceutical companies are struggling to create new structures to encompass translational research and yet are under considerable time pressure to generate innovation forced by the genericisation of the majority of high revenue cytotoxics by 2008.

As we move into a molecular target based future, cancer diagnostics will assume far greater importance in health-care delivery. Initial treatment decisions are currently based on skilled histopathology and imaging studies to determine the type, grade and stage of the tumour. To this may be added immunohistochemical assessment of hormonal receptor status and prognostic markers such as c-erbB2 expression. Yet histopathologists and their technical support staff are in short supply globally. This has driven increased laboratory automation at all stages from tissue handling through to image capture. Diagnostic strategies based on sophisticated tissue analysis are now poised to radically change cancer management from the identification of people with a high risk of developing cancer through to the precise prediction of toxicity of a specific drug in an individual. Despite the hype genomics, proteomics and other holistic strategies are too vague to be used to guide drug development decisions in practice today. The large number of variables creates a bioinformatic nightmare. Achieving the goal of personalised medicine for cancer will require a revolution in diagnostics and the dawn of a new era in tissue analysis through classical quantitative immunohistochemistry.

Molecular signatures

The traditional approach to cytotoxic drug development is not appropriate for many new agents for several reasons. Firstly, as their precise molecular mechanism is known it should be possible to develop a PD assay for their molecular effectiveness in patients. This can be used to determine the maximally effective dose for use in further studies. This approach will replace the classical phase I study which has in the past been used to evaluate the maximal tolerated dose. Although PD end points have been used for DNA binding drugs in the past, specific relevant assays were simply not available. Secondly, it may not be possible to rely on tumour response in phase II as a guide to survival benefit. Many of the new agents will cause disease stabilisation and not shrinkage. Thus, it will be necessary to commit to expensive randomised phase III studies without having the confidence generated by a successful phase II programme. The key to success in this mechanistically based future will be the collection of far more data in the early phase of drug development by the use of surrogates of both molecular target effects and clinical efficacy. Increasing emphasis on linking diagnostics to therapy will become an essential component of cancer drug development.

The holistic profiling of tumours using several technologies to determine its likely natural history and optimal therapy is possible. The beginnings of such correlations have been used in assays for the expression of specific gene products in increased, reduced or mutated form. Examples include erbB1, erbB2, ras, and p53. The emerging technologies of genomics, methylomics, proteomics, and metabonomics can produce enormous datasets to correlate with tumour behaviour patterns and response to different therapies. Although current data is fascinating, it will take several years before "personalised medicine" becomes a reality for the majority of cancer patients. The next decade will bring novel technologies in all these areas together with increasingly sophisticated bioinformatic tools. There is now a great need for ethically collected fresh tissue (both normal and malignant) to develop novel assays and determine variation. The new Human Tissue Authority in the UK is a welcome development, giving a well-defined legal framework for tissue donation after full consent.

A toolkit for early cancer drug development

The different components of an early development tool kit have different costs, risks and potential information yield. The investment payback will depend on how critical the information is to the successful development of drugs against a defined target. Thus, biomarkers of molecular effect are a requirement for all drugs. Surrogate end points of clinical benefit are particularly important for drugs whose long-term administration is necessary to achieve either tumour stabilisation such as anti-angiogenic or anti-invasive

<table>
<tr><td colspan="4" align="center">EGFR 1 and 2 as drug targets</td></tr>
<tr><td colspan="2">Small molecules</td><td colspan="2">Monoclonal antibodies</td></tr>
<tr><td>• Tarceva</td><td>Roche – OSI</td><td>• EMD72000</td><td>Merck</td></tr>
<tr><td>• EKB 569</td><td>Wyeth</td><td>• C225</td><td>Imclone – BMS</td></tr>
<tr><td>• PKI 166</td><td>Novartis</td><td>• Herceptin</td><td>Roche – Gen</td></tr>
<tr><td>• CI 1033</td><td>Pfizer</td><td>• MDX 210</td><td>Medarex</td></tr>
<tr><td>• Iressa</td><td>AZ</td><td>• Pertuzamab</td><td>Roche – Gen</td></tr>
<tr><td>• GW 2016</td><td>GSK</td><td>• DCC-E1A</td><td>Targeted gen</td></tr>
<tr><td>• TAK-165</td><td>Takeda</td><td>• Panitumomab</td><td>ABX</td></tr>
<tr><td>• AEE 788</td><td></td><td></td><td></td></tr>
</table>

Figure 7.5

agents where the cost in both time and effort of pivotal studies is immense. Success in achieving surrogate benefit here gives the confidence to commit long-term financial resource by effectively reducing the risk of failure and late stage attrition. Functional imaging studies are particularly helpful where optimising the effect of a drug requires precise scheduling – cell cycle inhibitors and pro-apoptotic agents. By obtaining real time images of mitosis and apoptosis in patients, logical decisions to enhance selectivity can be made more easily. Some biomarkers may well be surrogates for clinical efficacy under certain defined conditions. Biomarkers have different levels of specificity. Some can be used for a range of drugs affecting a biological process such as angiogenesis – others may be highly specific for the effects of a single agent. The toolkit therefore consists of a series of drawers containing generic assays for each category of a drug's action mechanism and a smaller compartment for the specific PD end point determination tools for an individual agent (Figures 7.5 and 7.6).

It currently takes an average of 10 years for a cancer drug to reach the market from the identification of the lead compound. The sheer number of potential cancer drugs now becoming available and the change of emphasis to targeted molecular mechanisms will require a rigorous selection process during the early phase of clinical development. Timelines will get shorter. Over the next decade systematic programmes of cancer risk assessment will be established and cancer preventive agents will enter into the clinic. Novel surrogate end points will be essential to determine their benefit without waiting for a further generation of cancer patients (Figure 7.7).

Creating a toolkit cancer drug development

	Cell cycle	Apoptosis	Signal transduction	Inflammation	Invasion	Angiogenesis	Differentiation
Biomarker	+	+	+	+	+	+	+
Surrogate				+	+	+	
Imaging	+	+				+	
Predictive signatures	+	+	+	+	+	+	+

Figure 7.6

Marketed targeted therapies

Drug	Generic	Manufacturer	Yearly cost (£ '000s)
Herceptin	Traztuzumab	Roche	60
Mabthera	Rituximab	Roche	40
Glivec	Imatinib	Novartis	50
Erbitux	Cetuximab	BMS	60
Avastin	Bevacizumab	Genentech	70
Tarceva	Erlotinib	Roche	65
Iressa	Gefitinib	AZ	40

Figure 7.7

Adapting to changing technology

One of the greatest challenges for an increasingly consolidated industry is to adapt to changing technology. The classical division of research departments into discovery and clinical is no longer optimal in this fast paced area. Drugs entering the clinic need to come with validated biomarkers of their PD effect, surrogates for clinical efficacy and a plan to stratify patients for likely response. Effective organisation of translational science is the key to the future and yet a significant challenge. Scientists are judged by the number of drugs getting out of the laboratory and into the clinic rather than how many are eventually brought to market and their commercial success. They are managed separately from clinical and experimental medicine groups. Clinical departments are concerned with operational excellence in the construction and execution of clinical trials. The drive to keep research and development costs down has resulted in cross therapeutic area sharing of emerging laboratory technology which can adversely influence close collaborative working. That a problem exists has clearly been recognised by most in senior management as demonstrated by the willingness of major oncology companies to experiment with their organisation.

As of 2001, a patient was entitled to about £20,000 worth of direct medical care cost for their cancer management. If we take a positive chemotherapy future, then by 2025, this figure could easily rise to £100,000 a patient per year – a total of perhaps £1 million over a lifetime.

Demand and supply of chemotherapy

We really have a cancer demand pyramid. In every society, rich and poor there is a core of services that are provided by the equivalent of the National Health Service (NHS) at the apex of the pyramid. There is a line that is wavy because of "post-code prescribing", above which there is demand but no payment. It is difficult to escape geographical variation with any localised decision-making input on resource rationing. Above the line, there are many unmet demands; complementary medicine, conformal radiotherapy, new drugs, new devices often heavily marketed to the end consumer through subtle techniques. The line is pushed down by NHS decision-makers; the regulators, National Institute for Clinical Excellence (NICE), hospital drug committees, primary care trusts, Strategic Health Authorities and politicians.

Possible scenarios for the future of chemotherapy

As we go into the future we simply do not know whether we are going to get technological success. So, there are four scenarios based on how successful we are and how much society is willing to pay:

1. The first is technological success and society somehow finding the costs to meet it, in which case cancer becomes a chronic controllable illness. That is obviously the preferred scenario for 2025.

2. The second scenario is where we achieve success but society is not willing to pay the cost. Then we get inequity and of course it will vary in different societies around the world. We can see this with human immunodeficiency virus (HIV) in Africa now.
3. If there is little technological success and if society is willing to pay, we will invest in supportive care.
4. The worst-case scenario is society not willing to pay and no technological success. We then have inequity in the distribution of supportive care and that is where cancer charities can lobby for the less fortunate to make sure that they actually get good supportive care.

Of course, no scenario leads to immortality. We do not like talking about death because we feel uncomfortable. No oncologist likes talking about death, in my experience this is because it is regarded as a sort of failure and most of us are even frightened to talk about our own mortality. Spending more money on supportive care in its broadest sense will be a good investment with all four possible futures. In reality, the future is probably somewhere in the middle. It is not going to work out well for every cancer, that is unlikely. The real future is somewhere in the middle, with bits from each scenario. The difficulty now for society is how to deal with this very uncertain future for chemotherapy. The crunch is going to come in 2008 when many of the drugs currently full of hope are scheduled for release onto the market and currently carry huge financial expectations of blockbuster success (Figure 7.8).

How does chemotherapy affect survival rates?

Very little improvement in survival has been achieved by the variations of the local control by permutations of radiation and surgery. Screening may have improved outcomes by shifting patients into earlier stages. We have also improved things by taking the assumption that many apparently localised cancers are actually advanced and treating them all with adjuvant systemic therapy. Intellectually, this is a shambles because we know that the gain from tamoxifen in breast cancer is at most around 15% of patients, so we are treating 85% of women with tamoxifen for nothing. So the first advance that is going to come out of proteomics and genomics is to use them to select which of localised cancers to leave well alone, after the loco-regional therapy. Personalised therapy is the key to the future.

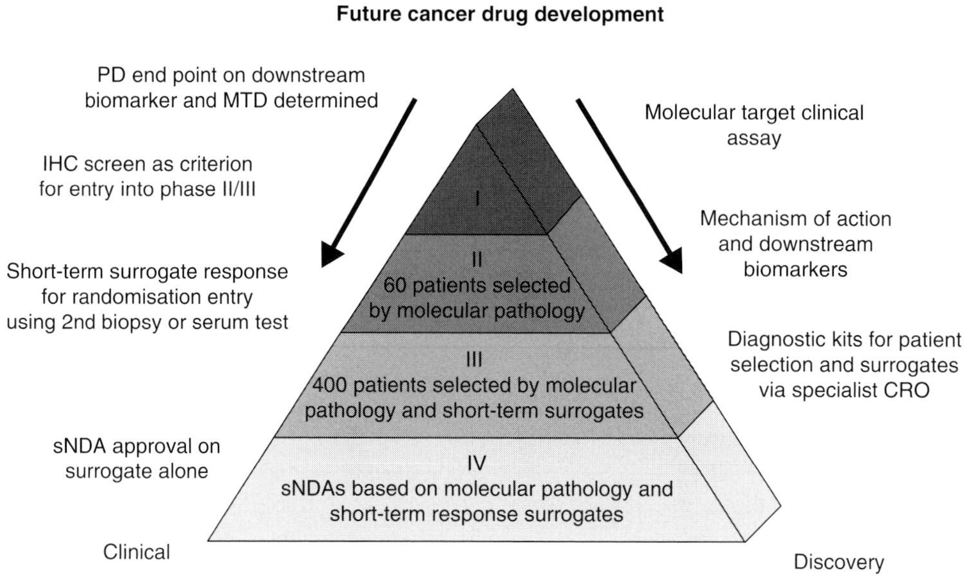

Future cancer drug development

PD end point on downstream
biomarker and MTD determined

IHC screen as criterion
for entry into phase II/III

Short-term surrogate response
for randomisation entry
using 2nd biopsy or serum test

sNDA approval on
surrogate alone

Clinical

Molecular target clinical
assay

Mechanism of action
and downstream
biomarkers

Diagnostic kits for patient
selection and surrogates
via specialist CRO

Discovery

I

II
60 patients selected
by molecular pathology

III
400 patients selected by molecular
pathology and short-term surrogates

IV
sNDAs based on molecular pathology and
short-term response surrogates

Figure 7.8

Predictions for evaluating the effectiveness of chemotherapies

Obviously one of the best ways to shorten the process of evaluating which characteristics in terms of gene and protein patterns are relevant to predict long-term success or failure is to get into archives where we know whether the patient has responded and is dead or alive 20 years later. The whole business of legislation on the protection of human rights and privacy could result in an uphill struggle for this kind of research. Dead people cannot give consent to their material being studied. We may have to concentrate much more on the use of surrogate end points and biomarkers, detected by imaging or repeat tumour biopsies. We have got to concertina our trials down so that we find more quickly how best to use this extraordinary technology. Pathology service companies are emerging who have recognised the need for properly consented tissue.

The Peterborough tissue bank was one of the first ethically consented tissue banks to collect prospectively for commercial drug development. A consent nurse sees the patient, explains the situation and gets a document signed that lawyers and the Department of Health are happy with. In the future, all cancer patients will be asked for such consent – it could actually benefit them

Cancer diagnostics in drug development

Diagnostic	Value
Predisposition screen	Identify patients for chemoprevention
Screen for presence of cancer	Increase in patients: earlier disease
PD biomarker	Establish pharmacological dose
Surrogate marker of clinical efficacy	Early indication of proof of concept
Predictive reclassification of disease	Target therapy to those likely to respond
Patient-specific toxicity prediction	Avoid adverse events, adjust dose

Figure 7.9

as well as others. When patients are approached with explicit information, 97% of them consent for their tissue to be used for whatever purpose so long as it is within a controlled governance framework. They even accept that it can be used for commercial gain. So the vast majority of the population actually wish to participate in this activity.

The importance of a systematic approach

We have defined a certain agenda for chemotherapy but surely there are other areas that are going to be very important between now and 2025? We are going to have more patients who have been treated with more powerful but selective agents and surely we need to get much more systematic monitoring using IT (Figure 7.9). The renal dialysis service has really set an example of how to do this systematically with every patient. They are measuring their urea levels, quality of life and so on. They have shown they can do it and we ought to be doing that in chemotherapy with all cancer drugs, new and old. If these scenarios are anywhere near correct then the population of cancer patients will stay stable or increase.

A global approach to chemotherapy delivery

The use of chemotherapy to treat cancer began in 1945, following the observation of leucopenia in military personnel exposed to mustard gas after an explosion of a battleship in Bari harbour. This alkylating agent was adapted for intravenous use and produced dramatic responses in patients with lymphoma and leukaemia. Other agents such as the folic acid and pyrimidine inhibitors rapidly followed and the armamentarium rapidly grew. It was recognised that drug resistance rapidly developed when single agents were used, so combination chemotherapy became standard. During the 1950s and 1960s, major strides were made in the treatment of leukaemias, lymphomas and choriocarcinomas with many patients becoming completely cured. New drugs were discovered following extensive screening programmes: the vinca alkaloids from the periwinkle, the anthracyclines from fungi and platinum drugs from experiments on the effects of electric currents on bacterial growth. The 1970s and 1980s brought effective drug combinations for testicular cancer and many childhood malignancies. The use of adjuvant chemotherapy for breast and colon cancer was proven to be beneficial in large scale randomised trials followed by sophisticated meta-analyses.

New drugs were launched and new combinations put together. For the last decade medical oncology has been on a plateau in terms of effectiveness (Figure 7.1). Despite many new agents becoming available, often at great cost, the gains in terms of cure rates have been small. Fashions for high dose chemotherapy with bone marrow transplantation, the use of marrow support factors, biological therapies such as monoclonal antibodies or cytokines have resulted in little overall gain at considerable expense. The driving force for medical oncology comes from the USA, which spends 60% of the world's cancer drug budget but has only 4% of its population (Figure 7.2). Huge cultural differences exist in the use of chemotherapy with US trained physicians following aggressive regimens for patients who in other countries would simply be offered palliative care. This has created a tremendous dilemma for those responsible for health-care budgets. The use of taxol in patients with metastatic breast cancer will prolong survival by 6 months but for a cost of $12,000. In many countries this would far exceed the total health-care consumption throughout a cancer patient's life. Yet the pressure to use expensive patented drugs is enormous. Conferences, travel, educational events sponsored by the drug industry rarely give a real perspective for effective prioritisation for poorer countries.

Delivery

Increasingly, chemotherapy can be given entirely in a day care setting. This reduces costs and is preferred by most patients and their families. Prior to initiation, the goal of therapy must be realistically defined. Prognostic factors such as the stage of the disease, the sites of metastases, the general medical condition of the patient, the willingness to accept any likely toxicity and the availability of the necessary facilities to treat complications must all be considered. Although a particular tumour may be curable in some circumstances, not all patients with that tumour type will be cured. The risk-benefit concept needs to discussed beforehand. Increasingly, cancer patients are being given more information about their disease and the options available. An honest appraisal of cost effectiveness is vital in countries where the full cost of drug is paid for by the patient. Cancer chemotherapy requires access to laboratory facilities to monitor at least blood counts, liver and renal function and basic circulating tumour markers. Nurse led chemotherapy suites are very effective and liked by patients. Clear protocols must be in place, adapted to local circumstance. The WHO essential anti-cancer drugs list is particularly helpful.

World Health Organisation (WHO) essential anti-cancer drugs list

Category 1	Category 2	Category 3
Bleomycin	Actinomycin D	Docetaxel
Chlorambucil	Busulphan	Erythropoietin
Cisplatin	Carboplatin	G-CSF, GM-CSF
Cyclophosphamide	CCNU	Gemcitabine
Dacarbazine	Cytarabine	Interferon – alpha
Doxorubicin	Daunorubicin	Irinotecan
5 fluorouracil	Mercaptopurine	LHRH agonists
Folinic acid		Paclitaxel
Etoposide		Topetecan
Methotrexate		Vinorelbine
Prednisolone		
Tamoxifen		
Vinblastine		
Vincristine		

The way forward

Cancer care in 2025 will be driven by the least invasive therapy consistent with long-term survival. Eradication, although still desirable, will no longer

> **Box 7.1: The uncertainty of novel drugs for cancer**
> 1. Will the new generation of small molecule kinase inhibitors really make a difference or just be expensive palliation?
> 2. How will big pharmas cope with most high value cytotoxics becoming generic by 2008?
> 3. Can expensive late stage attrition really be avoided in cancer drug development?
> 4. How will sophisticated molecular diagnostic services be provided?
> 5. Will effective surrogates for cancer preventive agents emerge?
> 6. Will patient choice involve cost considerations in guiding therapy?

be the primary aim of treatment. Cancers will be identified earlier and the disease process regulated in a similar way to chronic diseases such as diabetes. Surgery and radiotherapy will still have a role but this role may be downplayed. How much will depend on the type of cancer a patient has and the stage at which disease is identified. It will also depend on how well the drugs being developed today perform in the future and whether they are best used alone or in combination with these other interventions.

By 2025, cancer treatment will be shaped by a new generation of drugs. What this new generation will look like is not apparent in 2005 and will depend on the relative success of agents currently in development. Over the next 3–5 years, we will understand more fully what benefits these compounds such as the kinase inhibitors are likely to provide. It is estimated that in 2005 there were about 500 oncology drugs being tested in clinical trials. Of these, around 300 were against specific molecular targets. But this number is set to rise dramatically. Two thousand compounds will be available to enter clinical trials by 2006 and 5000 by 2010. Many of these drug candidates will be directed at the same molecular targets and industry is racing to screen those most likely to make it through in the development process. Tremendous pressures are coming from the loss of patent protection from the majority of high cost chemotherapy drugs by 2008 (Box 7.1). Unless new premium priced innovative drugs are available, cancer drug provision will come from global generic manufacturers currently gearing up for this change.

Future chemotherapy drugs

So what will these drug candidates look like? In 2005, small molecules are the main focus of research, most of which were designed to target specific gene products that control the biological processes associated with cancer such as signal transduction, angiogenesis, cell cycle control, apoptosis, inflammation, invasion and differentiation. Treatment strategies involving monoclonal antibodies, cancer vaccines and gene therapy are also being explored. Although we do not know exactly what these targeted chemotherapeutic agents will look like there is growing confidence that they will work. More uncertain is their overall efficacy at prolonging survival. Many could just provide very expensive palliation. In the future, advances will be driven more by biological understanding of the disease process.

Already we are seeing the emergence of drugs targeted at a molecular level – herceptin, directed at the human epidermal growth factor receptor 2 (HER2) protein, Glivec, which targets the Bcr-Abl tyrosine kinase, and Iressa and Tarceva, directed at epidermal growth factor receptor (EGFR) tyrosine kinase. These therapies, and others like them, will be used across a range of cancers. What will be important in 2025 is whether a person's cancer has particular biological or genetic characteristics. Traditional cancer categories will continue to be broken down and genetic profiling will enable treatment to be targeted at the right patients. Patients will understand that treatment options are dependent on their genetic profile. The risks and benefits of treatment will be much more predictable than today.

Selecting patients suitable for chemotherapy

Clinicians will have access to information that will help them recognise which localised cancers can be left alone and which tumours will respond to drugs. This will mean fewer patients being exposed to agents with unacceptable toxicity. Such predictive assays will dramatically improve the quality of life for cancer patients. Predictions will never be totally accurate and patients and doctors will still be faced with uncertainties. However, decisions will be better informed.

Therapies will emerge through our knowledge of the human genome and the use of sophisticated bioinformatics. Targeted imaging agents will be used to deliver therapy at screening or diagnosis. Monitoring cancer patients will also change as technology allows the disease process to be tracked much more closely. Treatment strategies will reflect this and drug resistance will become much more predictable. Biomarkers will allow those treating people with cancer to measure if a drug is working on its target. If it is not, an alternative treatment strategy will be sought. Tumour regression will become less important as clinicians look for molecular patterns of disease.

Preventive therapies

By 2025, there will be more of a focus on therapies designed to prevent cancer. A tangible risk indicator and risk reducing therapy, along the lines of cholesterol and statins, would allow people to monitor their risk and intervene. Delivering treatment early in the disease process will also be possible because subtle changes in cellular activity will be detectable. This will lead to less aggressive treatment. The role of pharmaceutical companies in the development of new therapies will continue to change. Smaller more specialised companies, such as those in the bio-tech sector, along with academia, will increasingly deliver drug candidates to the big pharmaceutical companies to market.

In 2025, people will be used to living with risk and will have much more knowledge about their propensity for disease. The IT infrastructure will be available for members of the public to determine their own predisposition to cancer. This in turn will encourage health-changing behaviour and will lead people to seek out information about the treatment options available to them. Patients will also be more involved in decision-making as medicine becomes more personalised. Indeed, doctors may find themselves directed by well-informed patients. This, and an environment in which patients are able to demonstrate choice, will help drive innovation towards those who will benefit. However, inequity based on education, wealth and access will continue.

Barriers to the introduction of new treatments

Innovation in cancer treatment is inevitable. However, there are certain prerequisites for the introduction of new therapies. First, innovation has to be translated into usable therapies. These therapies must be deliverable, to the right biological target, and to the right patient in a way that is acceptable by patient, health-care professional and society. Innovation must also be marketed successfully so that professionals, patients and those picking up the cost understand the potential benefits. Those making the investment in research will inevitably create a market for innovation even if the benefits achieved are small. The explosion of new therapies in cancer care is going to continue and pricing of these drugs will remain high. The cost of cancer drugs in 2005 is estimated to be $25 billion globally, of which $16 billion was spent in the USA. If effective drugs emerge from the research and development pipeline, the cancer drug market will be worth $300 billion globally by 2025, with this cost spread more equally to the rest of the world.

But parallel to this explosion in therapies and increase in costs, a number of confounding factors will make markets smaller. The technology will be there to reveal which patients will not respond to therapy so making block-buster drugs history. Doctors will know the precise stage of the disease process at which treatment is necessary. And as cancer transforms into a chronic disease, people will have more co-morbidities, which will bring associated drug–drug interactions and an increase in care requirements.

How do we balance this equation? The pharmaceutical companies will not necessarily want to do the studies to fragment their market. Research leading to rational rationing will need to be driven by the payers of health care. There is a risk that pharmaceutical companies will stop developing drugs for cancer and focus instead on therapeutic areas where there is less individual variation and therefore more scope for profit. Furthermore, development costs are rising. Ten years ago, the average cost of developing a new cancer drug was around $400 million: in 2005, it is nearly $1 billion. At this rate of growth, the cost of developing a new drug in 2025 could be $2 billion, an amount unsustainable in a shrinking market. With this in mind, the process of developing drugs needs to be made simpler and faster.

However, instead of research being made simpler, changes in legislation concerned with privacy and prior consent are making it more difficult. The European Union (EU) Clinical Trials Directive will make quick hypothesis testing trials impossible. Other challenges exist, as well, such as obtaining consent for new uses of existing human tissue – following political anxiety when consent for removing and storing tissues had not been obtained in the early years of the 21st century. However, surveys in 2003 have shown that patients who gave consent for tissue to be used for one purpose were happy for it to be used for another. They do not wish to be reminded of their cancer years later. To overcome these constraints regulators will have to start accepting surrogate markers rather than clinical outcomes when approving therapies. Outcome studies may well move to post-registration surveillance of a drug's efficacy similar to cholesterol lowering agents today.

Institutional barriers to new therapies

Other factors that will impact on the introduction of new therapies include dampeners such as the NICE or its equivalent in the early part of the 2020s. Assessing new technologies takes time, even for those with good evidence to support them. There will also be a battle for resources as cancer is transformed into a chronic disease. More people will be receiving prophylactic as well as long-term therapies. Even if these therapies turn out to be cheap, the numbers of patients involved and the monitoring diagnostics will mean overall costs will rise.

There will be a range of new players where firms emerge as key contributors. The last phase of oncology was dominated by a small number of firms with increased consolidation. The key contributors include:

• Bristol Myers Squibb
• Astra Zeneca
• Novartis
• Roche
• Eli Lilly
• Aventis.

The next phase will see the emergence of new players who succeed in developing new drugs. There are also signs of a geographic shift with little success being experienced by the US majors in their own research and development. European and especially Swiss companies and Japanese companies may well have a better success rate for innovation. For companies who develop new therapies there may be rewards in longer proof of exclusivity. Barriers to entry will include not just the original patent but manufacturing problems of more complex bio-tech drugs and the investment in diagnostics required to target the drugs successfully (Figure 7.10). Thus the industry faces a period of intense competition followed by the emergence of a new range of lead firms.

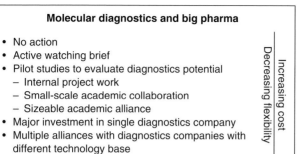

Figure 7.10

The drug industry will continue to compete for investment in a competitive, capitalist environment.

1. Personalised therapies are difficult for today's industry machine.
2. Surrogate end points will be essential to register new drugs.
3. Novel providers will emerge providing both diagnostic and therapy services.
4. Payers will rigidly seek justification for the use of high cost agents.

REFERENCES

1. Kleinke D. (2004) Think globally, protect locally: a conversation with Mark McClellan Health Affairs 23(3): 177–185.
2. Susman E. (2004) Accelerated approval seen as triumph and roadblock for cancer drugs. *Journal of the National Cancer Institute* 96(20): 1495–1496.
3. Bosanquet N. and Sikora K. (2004) The economics of cancer care in the UK. *Lancet Oncology* 5: 568–574.
4. Cancer Drug Predictions, McKinsey and Company, New York, 2001.

8

Moving towards the new model: international comparison

In this chapter we explore how different systems are moving towards the new model of cancer care. The USA has the best long-term data on changes in cancer care. The results there have been achieved in a pluralistic system. The UK presents an example of a highly centralised approach. Asia, on the other hand gives an example of a very limited response so far with an open field for future development.

USA

The services in the USA have been the pathfinders for world cancer services in terms of improving outcomes and changing models of care. The long-term data monitoring through Surveillance, Epidemiology and End-results (SEER) makes detailed analysis of outcomes and the effectiveness of care much more feasible than in most other health system. USA evidence has to be studied for its lessons for other systems. The USA has also seen the greatest commitment by government to the funding of research and improvement in cancer care through the National Cancer Institute (NCI). The principle economic developments, which can be identified in the USA, are both strategic and economic:

1. The focus of cancer strategy has shifted from concern with research for a "big bang" scientific breakthrough to application of the integrated model of cancer care from prevention through the extension of screening for early-stage cancer and palliative care for later-stage cancer. Inequities in access and treatment between white and African/Americans are also receiving much more attention.
2. US data have the most complete estimates of the disease burden for cancer. The first estimates were made in the mid-1980s.

Economic costs of all illnesses and cancer by type of cost: US, 1985

Type	All illnesses		Cancer		
	Amount ($million)	Per cent	Amount ($million)	Per cent	Per cent of all illnesses
Total	679,712	100.0	72,494	100.0	10.7
Direct	371,400	54.6	18,104	25.0	4.9
Indirect	308,312	45.4	54,390	75.0	17.6
Morbidity	80,850	11.9	7170	9.9	8.9
Mortality	227,462	33.5	47,220	65.1	20.8

Source: Brown and Hodgson, 1992.

At this stage the results showed that treatment costs were a relatively low proportion of the total cost. Mortality costs were high reflecting the large number of premature deaths especially from lung cancer. For 1985, cancer ranked as the leading cause of death in the 45–64 age group with 34.4% of the total. Since 1985 we can estimate that the pattern of costs has changed as follows:

- Reduction in lung cancer has changed mortality costs but they still remain high. Cancer was still the most important cause of life years lost with a total of 8.4 million life years lost compared with 7.8 million for heart disease and 7.0 million for all other causes. Mortality costs will be affected mainly by the changing incidence of lung cancer, which accounted for 2.3 million of the life years lost in 2001 far more than for any other kind of cancer.
- Morbidity costs have risen with increased prevalence/survival. Changes in insurance/Medicare have increased the share of out of pocket costs in this total.
- Treatment costs have been stable as a proportion of total health care spending.

Thus, in the first years after the War on Cancer, spending on cancer treatment rose as a proportion of the total: this increase was not sustained. The data show that the cancer treatment has been treating more patients with a constant share of spending. Some of the pressures towards spending on technology and new drugs have been offset by reductions in hospital stay and admissions

National cancer treatment expenditures in billions of dollars, 1963–1995

Year	Cancer treatment spending	Total health care spending	Per cent of total
1963	1.3	29.4	4.4
1972	3.9	78.0	5.0
1980	13.1	217.0	6.0
1985	18.1	376.4	4.8
1990	27.5	614.7	4.5
1995	41.2	879.3	4.7

Source: NCI.

made possible in part by new anti-emetic drugs. Total spending on cancer care has risen faster than direct treatment costs with increased spending on prevention and screening. In addition to the published estimates, which are due for up-dating from the NCI, it will be possible to make estimates of the total spending at each stage of the care process:
- Prevention
- Screening
- Treatment
- Surgery
- Radiotherapy
- Chemotherapy

There are also estimates for spending on specific types of cancer, which show differences in cost between cancer types.

Estimates of national expenditures for medical treatment for the 13 most common cancers

Type of cancer	Per cent of all new cancers	Expenditure (in $US, 1996)	Per cent of all expenditure	Average Medicare payment
Breast	18.2	5.4	13.1	9230
Colo-rectal	11.7	5.4	13.1	21,608
Lung	12.5	4.9	12.1	20,340
Prostate	13.6	4.6	11.3	8869

(*cont.*)

Table (*cont.*)

Type of cancer	Per cent of all new cancers	Expenditure (in $US, 1996)	Per cent of all expenditure	Average Medicare payment
Lymphoma	4.2	2.6	6.3	17,217
Bladder	4.0	1.7	4.2	10,770
Cervix	2.3	1.7	4.1	13,083
Head and Neck	3.3	1.6	4.0	14,788
Leukaemia	2.1	1.2	2.8	11,882
Ovary	1.7	1.5	3.7	32,340
Melanoma	5.2	0.7	1.7	3177
Pancreas	2.1	0.6	1.5	23,504
Oesophagus	0.9	0.4	0.9	25,886
All other	18.1	8.7	21.2	17,201
Total	100.0	41.0	100	

Source: NCI.

There have also been estimates of cancer spending on patients under 65 years, which could be compared with Medicare-based data on spending for older patients. These data show wide differences depending on the levels of insurance coverage for patients under 65 years.[1] They estimate that the cost of a government programme to cover all patients under 65 years would range from $30 to $41 billion.

For the non-US there are some clear pointers to the future from the US pattern of costs. Cancers with either a high initial cost (colo-rectal) or longer-term recurrent cost are likely to rise as proportions of the total. Increasing sub-specialisation is likely to raise total costs. The US data show that for many less common cancers spending fractions are higher than incidence. Cancer treatment has been relatively low cost in the past as a declining proportion of total expenditure being allocated over a rising total number of patients: but this position is likely to change in the future. More active development of new therapies for an increasing patient base will increase spending on cancer care much more rapidly. Cancer screening costs have risen from a low level 20 years ago to $10 billion or more, which represents 20–25% of spending on active treatment. US practice has combined increasing concentration of services for rarer surgical procedures on cancer with the development of ambulatory oncology centres for local access for more common cancers and procedures. The SEER database has allowed accurate identification of success rates in surgery. For removal of the pancreas the mortality rate in low-volume hospitals was double that of high-volume hospitals. Lung resection was also more likely to be successful in high-volume hospitals.

There is less research evidence on the performance of ambulatory care centres: but these centres have been able to achieve very rapid moves from symptoms to diagnosis to treatment (2 weeks or less). These centres have also had incentives to reduce hospital admissions, which have contributed to the US shift away from in-patient treatment. One centre attributed the change to increased use of anti-emetic drugs. "This has been a revolution, we have been able to treat twice as many patients as 10 years ago with virtually no hospital admissions."

In 2002, 7% of adults in the USA had been diagnosed with cancer, which accounted for at least 30% of premature life year lost. Against this background the actual use of health services is quite limited. Patients with cancer made 16 million visits to office-based physicians in 2002 (1.8% of all visits). They had 1.2 million hospital discharges or 3.5% of discharges. The number of discharges had fallen by 8.5% since 1994. Many of the admissions that did take place were by elderly patients, so that the average length of stay was higher than the average at 7.1 days compared to 4.9 days. Patients with cancer as a primary diagnosis were 5% of current patients for home health care and 5.8% of patients for nursing home care. More research is urgently needed on whether this ease of local access has assisted the improved outcomes found in the USA. The high level of outcomes is particularly remarkable given the lack of insurance coverage of 15–20% of the population, which in other areas of care leads to delays in access to treatment. The US evidence may also show how difficult it will be to achieve further improvements when survival has reached towards 90% for many early-stage cancers and from this perspective cancer was already becoming a survivable illness.

In addition to the successes with early-stage cancer, there are also some more specific successes to record:

1. A fall in the incidence of lung cancer among men. Lung cancer incidence rates among men declined by 1.8% a year from 1991 through to 2000 and death rates declined by 1.7% a year. By 2000, there were fewer patients diagnosed with lung cancer and fewer deaths compared with 1980. However, the incidence of lung cancer rose among women.
2. Improvements in cure and survival for children with cancer.

3. Improvements in cure for testicular cancer.

4. Reductions in incidence of stomach cancer.

For lung cancer the gains are mainly due to smoking cessation. For children's cancer and testicular cancer the gains would seem to be due to improved treatment. For stomach cancer the causes are mainly due to changes in diet over the last 50 years. Better food storage, cooking techniques and food supply have apparently reduced the carcinogens present in the gastric contents.

There is new evidence on the gains to screening. Screening programmes were evaluated in terms of the gains in numbers of cases detected: but it is now clear that possible later gains in survival through detection of disease at an earlier should be taken into account. Earlier estimates based just on gains in sensitivity are now inadequate. The US evidence allows tracking of the interactions between screening and treatment in ways which were not possible with early studies such as the Swedish Two Counties Study, which were carried out before there was evidence on the longer-term effects of treatment.

HMO-based data now allow evidence on the longer-term effects of screening. A retrospective study analysed persons detected with colo-rectal cancer from 1993 to 1999 in Group Health Cooperative, a large HMO in Washington State. Total health care costs were compared for screen-detected versus symptom-detected individuals. During this time 717 cancers were detected through screening and 206 cancers by symptoms.

"In the 3 months before diagnosis, total costs were $7436 for persons with screen-detected cancer compared to $10,042 for symptom-detected cancer; 53% of screen-detected cancers were at an early stage compared to 30% of symptom-detected cases. Overall, the cost for the screen-detected group was $22,639 in the 12 months after diagnosis compared to $29,471 for symptom-detected cancer."[2]

There are still questions, however, as to whether the US results are any better than those in other developed health systems. What is the record so far in terms of economic evidence? Has the USA bought better outcomes for patients with the distinctive scale and intensity of treatment? For coronary heart disease (CHD) treatment activism allied to lifestyle change seemed by the end of the 1990s to have created a clear pattern by which outcomes and survival were much better in the USA. Age-adjusted death rates for heart disease and stroke have fallen by 59% and 69%, respectively, since 1950: but even in breast cancer treatment, which has received more funding than other types of cancer, there was little difference in results in the USA compared with other advanced countries. Some direct evidence is now available from a special study carried out by the Organisation for Economic Co-operation and Development (OECD).[3]

Relative 5-year survival rates (%) breast cancer

	40–49 years	50–59 years	60–64 years	65–69 years	70–79 years	80+ years	All
Canada (Manitoba) 1985–1989	78.5	76.5	76.9	82.1	77.7	79.4	78.4
Canada (Ontario) 1985–1989	79.4	75.7	75.9	80.9	77.5	68.4	76.5
France 1985–1989	82.6	79.6	88.0	81.2	83.2	78.4	82.0
Italy 1985–1989	82.2	75.8	77.6	78.6	82.2	75.7	79.0
Japan 1992	90.5	85.9	86.3	n.a	81.4	76.4	84.9
Norway 1990–1994	80.5	79.2	75.2	79.8	74.1	76.6	77.9
Sweden 1989	81.0	79.0	88.0	n.a	85.0	73.0	82.2
UK (England) 1993–1995	79.5	81.7	77.5	n.a	69.6	53.0	74.1
US 1989–1995	82.6	82.5	84.7	n.a	82.7	n.a	83.8

Source: OECD, 2003.

The OECD study of international outcomes in breast cancer is detailed and thorough: it shows a similarity of results for younger patients across nations with the UK as an outlier for its poor results with older patients. The US survival rates are almost the same as for France and Sweden. Other evidence within the USA confirms that gains in improving outcomes in breast cancer have been slow. A study of patients with breast cancer treated at the MD Anderson Centre in Texas showed that there were some survival gains for patient with metastatic or later-stage cancer: but the rate of improvement seemed to be similar to or even slightly below that found in large-scale study of patients with metastatic at 20 cancer centres in France from 1980 to 1999: "Using statistical adjustment techniques, we estimate that there has been a reduction in risk of approximately 1% for each increasing year although the change was not statistically significant."[4] Overall, the improvement in breast cancer survival has averaged at 3% a year. Earlier detection with treatment of more disease has been the key variable.

A cost-effectiveness study of technological change in medicine concluded that for patients with heart attacks change in treatment costs of $10,000 had contributed to a year-on-year increase in life expectancy valued at $70,000. For breast cancer, a change in treatment costs of $20,000 had only brought about a 4-month increase in life expectancy valued at $20,000 so that technological change was neither beneficial nor harmful. In other areas such as the treatment of heart attack, low-birth weight infants and cataracts, the net benefits for additional treatment had ranged from $70–240,000.[5]

In summary, there are also some significant areas in the impact of cancer services:

1. There has been little progress in improving survival for patients with lung cancer.
2. There are still significant differences in outcomes (in the USA as in the UK) between social and ethnic groups. For all cancers in 2001, mortality was 25% higher for black Americans mainly reflecting poorer survival rather than higher incidence. The NCI is now concentrating much more development effort on these issues.
3. The long-term quality of life of cancer survivors is much poorer than was hoped for with 50% of long-term survivors recorded as having very poor quality of life.[6]

An official report in 2004 estimated there were 9.8 million cancer survivors in the USA in 2001.[7] The Report showed that:

- 64% of adults whose cancer is diagnosed today can expect to be living in 5 years time. Omitting lung cancer the percentage would rise to 80–90%.
- Breast cancer survivors make up the largest group of cancer survivors (22%) followed by prostate cancer survivors (17%) and colo-rectal cancer survivors (11%).
- The majority (61%) of cancer survivors are aged over 65 and cancer survivors are one in six in that age group. Thus, there are very significant new challenges in raising quality of life for longer-term survivors.

Conclusions

The US system presents as one in which there has been a great central success. For most types of cancer detected at an early stage, 5-year survival rates are 90%: but this success has created new kinds of disparity with slower improvement for certain groups of patients. The findings have implications for the future of targeted therapies. Can targeting make a difference for patients with poorer outcomes or will it simply add to the total costs of treating patients who would have survived anyway?

United Kingdom

During the last 5 years over £2 billion (US$3.8 billion) of extra money has been spent on cancer services – the biggest funding change for a single disease ever in the history of British medicine. We examine the effects on the quality of care that patients receive. The National Health Service (NHS) Cancer Plan was born out of major deficiencies going back three decades. Doing something for cancer became a political imperative with the publication of the Eurocare-2 study[8] showing Britain to be consistently low in the 5-year survival league table for several common cancers. From a list of glaring equipment deficits, staff shortages and gross inequity in use of high-cost anti-cancer drugs, the cancer plan created an infrastructure for change based on a classical public sector model.[9] Several hundred new administrative staff have been appointed to re-engineer the cancer patient's journey. But this has not been followed by an increase in clinical capacity because of critical staffing shortages and the lack of a uniform information technology platform. A review of the 34 cancer networks shows considerable variation of uptake of new monies for cancer with ten networks spending less than 80% and three less than 60% of their allocated funding.[10] The glow of political benediction has been subject to the decay factors of local inertia, divergences of priorities and the inability to resolve severe professional staff shortages. But patient expectation has risen dramatically.

The NHS Cancer Plan

The NHS Cancer Plan[11] identified the need for fast, convenient, high-quality care with patients at the centre. It set out the actions and milestones to deliver the fastest improvement anywhere in Europe within 5 years based on a massive injection of earmarked funding. It included three major commitments: to reduce smoking in lower socio-economic groups; to reduce the delay from urgent referral to the beginning of treatment to 2 months; and, to invest an extra £50 million in palliative care each year from 2004. It provides an excellent strategy to improve the quality of cancer care but has only partially fulfilled its ambitions.

Staff shortages are particularly severe in certain professions. Delays for radiotherapy of up to 3 months are common with some patients waiting 6 months because of a shortage of therapy radiographers. A study from Glasgow has shown that 21% of lung cancer patients became unsuitable for curative treatment during the wait for their therapy.[12] As radiotherapy becomes more precise the staff time required increases thereby escalating the problem. There is little evidence of increased throughput in universities training radiographers and the loss from such degree programmes still exceeds 30%. Although there has been a rise in training numbers of oncology specialist registrars, consultant early retirement has increased significantly. In addition, there are many new demands on consultants' time from multidisciplinary team attendance, appraisal and accreditation as well as longer consultations. In some specialities critical for good cancer care the situation is actually deteriorating with the estimate of 400, a third of the total, vacant histopathology posts by 2005.[13]

Much acclaim has been given to the achievement of the 2-week target from urgent general practitioner (GP) referral to specialist consultation. There is little evidence to suggest that prior to 2000 this was a serious issue despite public statements to the contrary by Ministers.[14] There have been significant improvements in co-ordination that have been welcomed by patients. One-stop clinics for breast and other cancers reduce the anxiety associated with not knowing the detailed treatment plan for several weeks. Such initiatives depend on local enthusiasm as much as central directives and most were underway before the cancer plan was written.

Perhaps the biggest disappointment has been the inability to reduce the waiting period from referral or diagnosis to first treatment, except for breast cancer. This is due to simple under-capacity and shortage of critical staff. No amount of re-engineering can overcome these fundamental problems. Breast cancer is an exception because definitive treatment is excision biopsy for most patients. Surgeons were already adopting a far more streamlined approach to managing cancer patients stimulated by the success of their voluntary national audit system.[15] Radiotherapy and chemotherapy are not usually the first definitive treatments for breast cancer so delays here are simply excluded from the statistics.

Waiting time target data taken from the Department of Health web site[16] shows that there is a consistent lack of improvement for several types of cancer throughout 2002, almost certainly the result of under-capacity. The last posting of this electronically collected dataset is now 8-month old whereas last year results were posted monthly. This suggests a reticence to reveal more recent data. The target itself – a wait of 2 months from referral to first treatment – would be unacceptably long in most European countries and result in litigation in the USA.

The future context: new technology in cancer care

We are entering a period of rapid change in therapies with great potential for helping cancer patients. The plan has to aim at a moving target to satisfy an increasingly informed and medically sophisticated public. Surgery still remains the single most effective modality for cancer treatment. It is increasingly conservative, able to retain organs and structures. New technology permits minimally invasive surgery for many cancer types. Increased day-case work, less use of intensive care and fewer beds will reduce costs. The separation of diagnostic from emergency surgery through the creation of 44 privately run, NHS funded, diagnostic and treatment centres will reduce delay in cancer surgery.

Modern linear accelerators allow dose delivery to the precise shape of the tumour. Whilst 56 linear accelerators have been purchased with lottery funding, most have been replacement machines.[17] The effect of this initiative on waiting times has been dwarfed by radiographer shortages leading to temporary closures of existing machines. Conformal therapy aims to deliver high dose just to the tumour volume, killing the cancer cells and avoiding normal surrounding tissue. Equipment costs have doubled over the last 10 years and precision therapy has dramatically increased staffing requirements. As US practice has demonstrated, patients will seek out centres that can provide them with radical radiotherapy, which has less unpleasant long-term side effects.

Over the last 5 years there has been a shift away from the search for new cytotoxics to drugs acting on defined molecular mechanisms. Nearly 500 molecules are currently undergoing clinical study.[18] Britain is consistently low in its use of chemotherapy compared to other European countries. The correction of this deficit at a time of technological turbulence will create increasing financial pressure. The well-informed patient will seek guidance from emerging Internet second opinion services linked to global pharmacies for innovative drugs. The elimination of post-code prescribing for cancer drugs was a clear political imperative. Although reviews by the National Institute for Clinical Excellence (NICE) have been assiduously carried out and an extra £124 million spent on drugs, there are still reports of diversity in policies in NHS centres and purchasers.[19] The nationally agreed diagnostic process to assess women for trastuzumab for breast cancer is simply unavailable in some areas creating a novel form of rationing.

Key issues in cancer care delivery

Patients are demanding fuller information on treatment options. They will seek to follow the consumer trend of greater choice. As survival improves cancer will become a much longer-term, chronic illness. A higher proportion of sufferers will be elderly with problems of travelling for repeated episodes of treatment. Better information technology will make it possible to move towards more flexibility in local follow up.

Increasing numbers of oncologists will be frustrated if they are not able to increase activity or quality. More staff means that more patients can be treated or that the same numbers can be treated with higher quality. But inefficiencies in re-engineering may mean it is difficult to do either. Developing alternative models of care within the NHS for chronic illness is notoriously difficult. One area where there has been real success in improving both the quality and access are services for end-stage renal failure.[20] Annual demand for these services has been increasing at 5.3% per year since 1997. Hub-and-spoke models have been developed and patients now visit local satellite units with continuous, consistent monitoring of each patient through a national IT system.

Drivers of the new agenda

The requirement for funding is set to rise sharply as the underlying changes in technology impact on services. Earlier referral means more demands on diagnostics and more time on therapy. More intensive treatment for several advanced cancers is now mandated by NICE recommendation.[21] Improved overall survival partly results from more effective therapies but also shifts in the cancer profile away from lung and towards prostate. The result is likely to be a substantial increase in cancer prevalence.

For these reasons, we need programmes to improve quality of life and minimise recurrence risk. There is evidence that earlier intervention can reduce treatment costs. Simple surgical treatment of early oral cancer costs an average of £244 per patient whilst therapy for advanced disease costs over £4800 even at 1993 prices.[22] A study of Medicare patients with colo-rectal cancer showed costs were four times higher for more advanced disease than for early stages.[23] The recent report of the National Cancer Control Initiative in Australia has stressed the urgency of greater integration of care and has also shown how improvements in efficiency can be made at low cost. UK cancer networks will have to define how they might invest in order to minimise later costs.

The next decade

There is little discussion of efficiency in the Cancer Plan. The Cancer Collaboratives are currently working in an economic Garden of Eden, which must transform into a world where managers seek best value from limited funding. This needs an engine of economic incentives as well as laudable aspirations. Without new initiatives we cannot achieve a service aiming for access in days not months. The issue of productivity is central to achieving targets. Re-engineering without incentives will not improve overall outcomes.

The gap between potential services and their funding is widening. Cancer treatment should have the same principles of choice and variety of providers that are being offered in other areas of health care. Its inclusion in national tariffs will allow the relative costs of different providers to be dissected. Diagnostics and radiotherapy would be good pilots for a choice programme so that patients get an alternative service if there are delays. Unless there are increased opportunities for innovation there will be a tilt of health investment into other areas and cancer care will become disadvantaged yet again.

Significant improvements in access and capacity over the next 2 years are essential to take the momentum forward. Local initiatives could raise productivity by 20% in cancer centres. A range of providers should be encouraged through open tendering so as to end the block on investment and innovation. We need to improve the information available to patients on quality and access. But short-term vote attracting initiatives by politicians must be separated from the sustainable development of cancer services.

Summary points

- Local initiatives to raise productivity by 20% in cancer centres over the next 2 years are urgently needed.
- National tariffs for key modules of cancer care will allow comparison between different providers and drive efficiency.
- The patient choice system should be extended to cancer treatment together with improved public information on quality and access.
- Private sector involvement through open tendering will end the block on investment, innovation and imaginative human resource policies.
- A single national IT platform for cancer care should allow more efficient use of resources delivered by private and public providers.

Asia

Asia has a massive challenge in using the staged model to reduce the likely rise in mortality from cancer. We carried out a systematic review of national and international evidence on health funding and patterns of health service. We also review forecasts of disease patterns and economic change in Asia from WHO, The World Bank and non-governmental sources. We seek to compare results for Asia with those in Europe and the USA. There may have been health policy convergence across the North Atlantic but such convergence has not been the pattern between Asia and Europe.

Health spending as a proportion of gross domestic product (GDP) has not increased in line with economic development. In Asia, the share of GDP spent on health has not increased in relative terms even though it has risen in absolute terms. The overall average is low, which for some countries can be explained by their low level of real income. For example, European/US parameters show an income elasticity for health spending of at least 1. In order to reach that level, health spending in Malaysia would be 5–6% of GDP rather than the actual figure of 2.5%. Moreover, even higher spenders such as Japan and Korea are well below the 10–14% found in France, Germany and the USA.

Private, out of pocket spending is much higher than the 10–20% found in Europe. With the exception of Japan, which in this respect shows a more European pattern, private out of pocket health expenditure ranges from 41% in the Republic of Korea to 82.2% in India. The main growth in health services in the past 10 years has been in private services. These are particularly likely to be used by patients from lower-income groups while access to the public sector is mainly confined to public employees and those with special privileges. The availability of medical staff is much lower than in Europe. For example, Malaysia had 65.8 physicians per 100,000 population in 1997 (the most recently available figures) while Germany had 350. The hospital bed/population ratio is only half, or less than half in main Asian countries than in Europe and the USA. Asian health systems score poorly (apart from Japan and Singapore) on WHO criteria of quality.

Currently there is substantial early mortality and high costs from disease in much of Asia. Against this background of severe limitations in resources Asia faces steep increases in disease prevalence. Our review of available forecasts shows particularly steep increases in cancer. WHO estimates show that there were 10.1 million new cases of cancer in 2000: by 2020 the number of new cancer cases will increase to 15 million. Over the course of a decade nearly 3% of the world's population will be diagnosed with cancer. Total prevalence will increase even more than this with improved survival. For Asia there will be a unique challenge. At present, patterns of cancer are very different from Europe with a high incidence of cancers related to infections.

Incidence of cancer in Western Europe and Eastern Asia, 2000

Type of cancer	Western Europe		Eastern Asia	
	Men	Women	Men	Women
Stomach	13.8	7.0	42.6	19.6
Lung	53.2	10.7	39.4	15.0
Liver	Low	Low	35.5	12.7
Colo-rectal	42.1	29.4	17.8	12.5
Breast	–	78.2	–	18.1

Age standardised rates per 100,000 population.
Source: WHO, 2003.

For example, chronic carriers of Hepatitis B are much more likely to contract cancer of the liver. There are also special lifestyle problems such as the effects of long-term exposure to cooking fumes, which cause lung cancer for women in China. Asia faces a situation where there may be both an increase in developed country cancers among more affluent people along with a continued high level of other cancers in rural areas. In addition to the impacts of an increasing (India) and ageing (China) population, there is likely to be further changes which will mean that the number of new cases of cancer will rise faster than the predicted global average.

Scenarios for Health Services in Asia

We can assess the likely changes in main variables affecting demand and supply.

Demand is likely to be determined by:

- the rate of growth of real incomes;
- changes in disease patterns, which could influence both total demand and its composition between product types;
- changes in customer/patient expectations.

Supply will be determined:

- by market growth;
- sources of funding/insurer/private/government;
- company development and strategy.

Growth rates of real incomes are likely to continue at 8–10% across much of Asia. In effect, average incomes are likely to double over the next 10 years for India and China. These countries are also at the level of income where they are likely to show higher income elasticity of spending for health care. Thus, the next 10 years are likely to show expansion of health spending at similar rates to those of the Republic of Korea in the last decade.

The growth of real incomes is likely to lead to greater service differentiation in the health care market. There will be an increase in high-value services based on hospitals and polyclinics funded by employer-based insurance schemes. There may be some internationalisation of this market with cheaper air travel and greater availability of information through the Internet with the development of special centres in the free zones of the Gulf States and in India. The successful model of Emirates Airline may be replicated in the newly developing Dubai Health Care City. There will also be a large increase in services for a self-pay market which will expand and will show greater diversity from specialised clinics and treatment centres through to more local services associated with community pharmacies.

Governments are likely to come under pressure to develop a more active role in countering infectious disease and other threats to public health. There will be an increasing market for products and services, which will be used in such endeavours. These will be partly funded by private foundation and special international funds. There is likely to be an increase in the market for turnkey programmes for delivering service to the population as well as for specific products such as vaccines.

Supply will be affected by the relative size of the markets for high-tech equipment and for the middle self-pay market. Our perspective is that the market for hospital-based high-tech equipment will remain relatively small as Asia will continue to depend less on hospital service than Europe, the USA or even Latin America. There is likely to be much more international competition with the emergence of specialised wholesalers and more entry by international firms. Price trends will be highly variable – some types of product will become commodities with strong downward pressure on prices: for others stronger branding and marketing will led to greater price stability. Supply will be greatly affected by company strategies and by entry into the field. Will larger Asian companies with a strong position in electronics and global markets leverage their brand names in this field? Compared with markets for consumer products the markets for diagnostics/medical devices are very fragmented. But there could be opportunities for companies to use their expertise in product development for products and services, which are related to the specific requirements of markets in Asia. It may also be that international companies from the USA and Europe will develop more specific capability in Asia.

Thus, within Asia the most important variables affecting companies are likely to be health specific, with the general economic rate of growth as a background factor that is unlikely to change significantly any developments in the market. To an exceptional extent, the outcome will be affected by company strategy and entry. The fundamental question will be whether the health care industries of Asia become as central to the future Asian economy as such companies have been in Europe and the USA? Much will depend on whether there is a new momentum of innovation and product development.

Possible scenarios

We can distinguish between two possible scenarios:

1. At one extreme, there is a scenario in which limited resources are stretched across a rising range of serious health problems. There are increasing social and economic losses as a result of poor access to treatment, which is often only available as a last resort on an emergency basis rather than early in the disease process as a preventative measure. There is a continuing shortage of staff, which is intensified by movement of qualified staff towards Europe and the USA.

2. In a more benign scenario, the Asian health economy shows a rapid and flexible response to new challenges. Additional services will develop in smaller hospitals/clinics rather than in large hospital hubs. The market for medical devices/diagnostics will grow rapidly through a range of small- to medium-ticket items rather than through big-ticket hospital-based items with greater similarity to consumer markets. There will be new synergies with lifestyle and communication products in services such as hearing aids. There will be innovative ways of financing equipment through rental or leasing. Innovation will be in equipment for short-stay and day treatment, and in use of the Web. Community pharmacies will also play a major role in developing the markets for diagnostics/bandages/wound dressings and smaller equipment.

Company strategies

One key variable will be the response of companies in supplying the wide range of goods and services to Asian patients and health professionals. We now examine the key choices facing companies and their impact on the market.[24] The strategies of Asian companies have to be seen against a background of rapid change in markets for imaging/devices/diagnostics. The imaging industry has seen increasing consolidation with Siemens, General Electric and Toshiba as the leaders. General Electric remains the world leader but is now facing greater challenge from Siemens, which has developed a new strategy of providing a total service with a strong IT element. It has made a significant acquisition in the USA of SMS (Shared Medical Systems), which are a leading US supplier and developer of IT for the health care sector.

The imaging industry has concentrated thus far on the market for large equipment in big hospitals in the USA and Europe. This market, however, is declining in Europe. In Europe, the largest market is in Germany where hospital investment declined 17% in real terms from 1991 to 2001. In the future, the industry may have to concentrate more on developing equipment or smaller hospitals and clinics. There may be a similar transition to that in the aircraft industry where demand for smaller regional jets from newer producers such as Bombardier and Embraer is rising much faster than demand for larger aircraft.

Such development is likely to increase the potential for remote image interpretation. Such a market has already developed between India and the USA in radiology and is likely to be the first step towards much more international transmission and trade in services. The devices/diagnostics industry is shifting away from the older model of family run firms towards greater leadership by a few research-based firms. The leaders include Johnson and Johnson, Roche, Becton Dickinson, and Smith and Nephew. Smith and Nephew provides an example of strategic decision-making as it has divested many activities to concentrate on three main areas: orthopaedic implants, wound care and surgical equipment, and has shifted away from product areas such as OTC Medication and rehabilitation equipment where returns were lower.

There are also newer entrants who grew rapidly in a specific product area – coronary transplants or laser adjustment of vision. These face a much shorter product life cycle leading to greater price competition. The first wave of innovation starting in the 1980s, associated with names such as Boston Scientific and Medtronic, was mainly for products used in a hospital setting. The new wave of innovation is more related to patient testing in primary and ambulatory care. We would also signal one important area of international convergence – this is the development of chains of community pharmacies. There has been a great deal of consolidation in the UK where the three main chains now control over 50% of pharmacies: new types of pharmacy business have begun to emerge in Asia and in Latin America with the growth of Apollo in India and Farmacias Ahumada in Chile/Peru and Brazil.

Future opportunities

Our results point to significant growth opportunities for regional producers as well as for established international companies. There will be opportunities for companies with experience in consumer markets to develop in these sectors. Companies can work with a new generation of physicians to develop ambulatory care/clinics and extended primary care. Much of the new requirement for treatment will involve long-term care of chronic illness: diabetes, CHD and preventive care after a first episode of cancer. This will require improvements in the diagnostic capability, disease monitoring and treatment.

There will be scope for much wider use of IT. The key issue for Asia is that of improving the capability and productivity of health professionals to deal with the huge challenges over the next decade. Local studies have been positive about the potential for the private sector to develop services even in poorer areas. Local physician practices can play a much-expanded role through health teams and through building networks for more specialist care. Key areas for development in ambulatory/community care would include:

1. Development of local health check and screening programmes.
2. Diagnostic testing and care programme design.
3. Delivery and monitoring of therapies.

There is a middle area between primary and hospital care, which is currently tilted by tradition and capital investment towards hospital services. The development of IT involving much easier access to evidence and care programme, and much easier transmission of test results makes it possible to reclaim much of this middle area for new kinds of ambulatory care. Even within developed country health systems there have been examples of very strong shifts away from hospitals in various types of care. Asia now has the opportunity to fill the development gap through developing much more intensive services which are not attached to hospital in-patient care.

The Community Pharmacy can play a much larger role in improving access to services. The last decade has seen a new range of effective drug therapies. Pharmacies can play a vital role in ensuring that patients can gain access to a wide range of new drugs. This can also promote the market for high-quality generics as well as for brand name drugs. Community pharmacies can also play an important role in providing monitoring, special diets and support for patients with long-term illness such as CHD and diabetes. There are a number of ways in which pharmacies can offer partnership and support to customers in high-risk groups. This could involve a range of products or lifestyle change, health monitoring and exercise/diet programmes. Marketing could be by web sites and text messages as well as by direct contact.

Community Pharmacies can also act as hubs or local health specialists and support services.

The role of Community Pharmacies is especially relevant where there is no "cradle to grave" welfare state so that people need quick access to services for rapid recuperation and health maintenance. Most of the costs of ill health in Asia are born by patients and carers themselves: and ill health leads directly to loss of earning power and falling living standards. Thus services that improve access for the mass market of self-pay patients will be particularly important.

The growth of the new Asian ambulatory care and the extended role of community pharmacies would enlarge the markets for a wide range of products and services in areas such as diagnostic equipment, wound care products and pharmaceuticals. The market could develop strongly but in very different ways from that in Europe. Asia in effect has the chance to use its expertise in IT and electronics to catch up. Asia can jump an evolutionary stage in health care. It can move directly to the stage of integrated care with much more use of networks and distance diagnosis. It will certainly need to make this evolutionary leap if there is to be any chance of meeting the new challenges faced by health care in Asia.

Summary

In different ways in all these situations we see new responses to public and professional demands. The new model of cancer is emerging with much more emphasis on prevention and screening, and new kinds of ambulatory care centre. In the final section we set out a feasible, fundable model for making full use of the new-staged model of cancer care.

REFERENCES

1. Thorpe K. and Howard D. (2003) Health insurance and spending among cancer patients. *Health Affairs*, April 2003, 1–6.
2. Ramsey S.D. et al. (2003) Cancer-attributable costs of diagnosis and care for persons with screen-detected versus symptom-detected colorectal cancer. *Gastroenterology* 125(6): 1645–1650.
3. OECD (2003) A Disease-Based Comparison of Health Systems. OECD Paris.
4. Giordano S. et al. Is breast cancer survival improving? *Cancer* 100(1): 44–52.

5. Cutler D. and McClellan M. (2001) Is technological change worth it? *Health Affairs* 20: 11–29.

6. Yabroff K.R. et al. (2004) Burden of illness in cancer survivors. Findings from a population-based national sample. *Journal of the National Cancer Institute* 96(17): 1322–1330.

7. CDC (2004) Cancer Survivorship – United States 1971–2001. In: Mortality and Morbidity Weekly Report. June 25.

8. Berrino F., Capocaccia R., Esteve J. et al. Survival of cancer patients in Europe. *The EUROCARE – 2*: IARC Scientific Publications No 151, Lyon, France 1999.

9. Kunkler I. (2000) Managed clinical networks: a new paradigm for clinical medicine *Journal of the Royal College of Physicians* 34: 230–233.

10. Richards M. *Investment in Cancer in 2001/2002 and 2002/2003* Department of Health, London.

11. *The NHS Cancer Plan* (2000) Department of Health, London.

12. O'Rourke N. and Edwards. (2000) Lung cancer waiting times and tumour growth *Clinical Oncology* 12: 141–144.

13. Royal College of Pathologists Submission to NICE on liquid based cytology for cervical screening. RCP, London, 2002.

14. Hutton J. Today Programme, BBC 4, 26th May 2003 http://news.bbc. co.uk/1/hi/health/2937552.stm

15. Patel R., Smith D. and Reid I. (2000) One-stop breast clinics – victims of their own success? A prospective audit of referrals to a specialist breast clinic. *European Journal of Surgical Oncology* 26: 452–454.

16. www.modern.nhs.uk/cancer Cancer Services Collaborative, National Monthly Progress Reports.

17. *New Opportunities Fund* Department of Health, London (1999).

18. Sikora K. (2002) Surrogate endpoints in cancer drug development. *Drug Discovery Today* 7: 951–956.

19. Editorial Another NICE Mess (2002) *Lancet Oncology* 3: 385.

20. UK Renal Registry Report 2002.

21. Delivering the NHS Plan Expenditure Report, Department of Health, London 2003.

22. Downer M. (1998) An interim determination of health gain from oral cancer and precancer screening. *Community Dental Health* 15: 72–76.

23. Brown M., Riley G. and Potosky A. (1999) Obtaining long-term disease specific costs of care application to medicare enroles diagnosed with colo-rectal cancer. *Medical Care* 37: 1249–1259.

24. Atun S., Shah S. and Bosanquet N. (2002) The medical devices sector: coming out of the shadow. *European Business Journal* 14(2): 63–72.

9

The new agenda

We have sought to set out the challenges to the teams who make cancer services across the world. In each nation there are few key decision makers and agents of change. They now have to face up to a new agenda. At first sight there might seem to be some rather major indeed insuperable difficulties in the way of continued progress in the twin aims of improving outcomes and quality of life. In developed countries we are already achieving 90% survival rates for most early stage cancers. There has already been a considerable expansion in screening, which has produced very clear results in cancer of the cervix, and access to chemotherapy has improved. The World Cancer Report left an abiding impression of the sheer scale of the problem with mortality of 2 m a year in developed countries and 6 m worldwide. On estimates for the US, 46% of men and 36% of women will be diagnosed with cancer in the course of their lives and improved survival will produce a doubling in prevalence.

We can identify two possible scenarios. In one, we use limited resources in an effective way to achieve key aims within the model of staged cancer services. There is an alternative scenario in which we simply muddle on through expanding the current disconnected modules of service.

Effective use of resources within the model of staged cancer services

The international evidence is that a number of key actions can make a real difference to mortality in developed countries. Research and international service development over the last two decades have shown that the following actions are likely to be effective:

- *Prevention through smoking cessation*: If we aim for a 20% reduction in total mortality in developed countries and 40% in premature mortality then reductions in smoking rates are vital. Based on the existing evidence, there are no other ways that such targets are going to be reached.

- *Targeted screening*: Selective expansion of screening programmes on a population basis can assist earlier detection both directly and indirectly through raising awareness more widely of the importance of early diagnosis.
- *Developing one stop ambulatory cancer centres*: The international evidence from the US points to effective results if there can be a maximum of 2 weeks for diagnosis and treatment. Most cancer patients in the UK and in Europe are taking months to move through the patient pathway. Speed in the diagnosis/treatment process certainly contributes to favourable outcomes in the US, and it also reduces the cost of treatment. Current services outside the US are based on high levels of hospital admissions and lengths of stay for cancer patients. With less invasive surgery and the availability of anti-emetics, such high levels of lengthy stay hospital admissions in early stage cancer are quite wasteful. There is a worldwide challenge of freeing up resources from hospital treatment to fund more intensive treatment.
- *Activism works*: More intensive chemotherapy and radiotherapy (sometimes in combinations) improve survival. Again the use of anti-emetics has reduced side effects for patients. Activism is also important in monitoring and treating recurrence.
- *Patient experience*: The patient's experience can and must be improved through improved communication, increasing access to complementary therapies and better palliative care.

Muddling through disconnected modules of service

The alternative scenario is that we simply muddle on through expanding the current disconnected modules of service:

- there is a failure to achieve key targets in prevention so that mortality from lung cancer continues to be high;
- screening increases mainly through repeated opportunistic screening of people in low-risk groups while full population coverage is not achieved;
- the treatment process is slow and fragmented and there is a multiplication of high-cost capital equipment in a few big cities;
- there are differences in access to new high-cost therapies and under use of effective generics;
- although survival improves many survivors have high level of disability and a poor quality of life;

- there is shortage of palliative care and poor access to morphine;
- lastly, the aim of privacy, dignity and control in the last phase of life is not achieved.

Which scenario will it be?

We have it in our power to bring about the first scenario. In developed countries there will have to be a very significant re-engineering of services to achieve the aims. In middle-income countries there can be a catching up so that they can raise 70% survival rates to 90%. They can also make great gains in prevention. In this chapter we set out feasible and fundable changes that could move cancer services forward. Successful change does not require large amounts of new spending or high-cost capita. We need a one-off investment in the new staged model of care followed by steady development over a period of years.

However, we can be far clearer on how the staged model of cancer services can be implemented. It has to start from an appreciation of feasible options, based upon an emerging model of international best practice. This includes:

1. national cancer strategies,
2. new integrated cancer programmes,
3. screening,
4. early detection and treatment,
5. follow-up and secondary prevention,
6. palliative care.

Accepting likely constraints of funding and to the structure means there can still be movement towards the model so as to achieve improved outcomes, reduce disease burdens and make progress, even with anticipated fiscal strains.

Figure 9.1 shows schematically the complex range of components and their relationships, which make up a modern national cancer plan. The need to develop and refine, such holistic models as a basis for consensus building and investment planning is now gaining recognition with key contributions from the National Cancer Institute (NCI) in the US Scandinavia, and more recently the UK. This type of model replaces older ones, in which cancer treatment is seen as matter of an individual clinician waiting for patients to bring in symptoms. It involves a cancer strategy, which seeks to maximise prevention, early detection, effective treatment and follow on care involving management of risk and/or palliative care. This new approach rests on an evidence base that has been greatly strengthened and enlarged over the last 10 years.

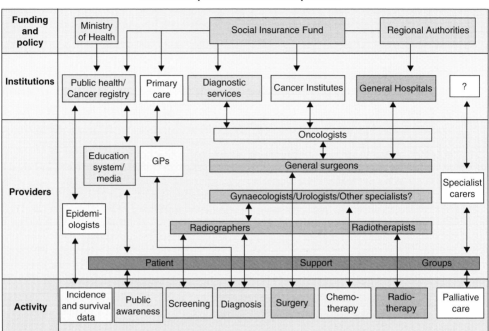

Figure 9.1   Cancer prevention and care process.

Prevention

Here there is firm evidence on the immediate results in smoking prevention in reducing lung cancer from the UK and the US. Poland adopted strong policies to reduce smoking in the early 1990s. By 2000, the incidence of lung cancer had fallen, while it had shown no change in Hungary and the Czech Republic.

Changes in diet

Changes in diet towards eating more fruit and vegetables will also have helped to reduce cancer incidence. Any increase in obesity will strengthen a risk factor.

Early detection

The vital role of screening programmes is already recognised, most notably for cervical cancer, and to a lesser extent for breast cancer. Survival is related strongly to stage of diagnosis for most cancers and gains in survival have been driven by earlier detection. Countries or insurance funds with the strongest gains in survival have been most active in introducing and extending screening programmes.

Use of protocols/care pathways

With the development of chemotherapy and radiotherapy, there are now an increasing number of options and combinations for treatment. At the same time, the diagnostic process is becoming more complex. To meet clinical governance standards cancer centres are using protocols and care pathways. This is driving new investment in information technology.

Drug therapies

Optimal use of the ever-expanding range of drug therapies: and targeting therapies for best results for patients.

Improved communication with patients

Increasingly patients are seeking to be involved in decision-making and want to have the options discussed with them.

Use of multi-disciplinary teams

The practice of regular team meetings to discuss patients involving surgeons, radiotherapists and oncologists is now being used much more widely, adding to the pressures for improving the information base.

Specialist nurses

Specialist nurses are increasingly being seen as key team members in managing treatment programs and communicating with patients.

The development of follow-up and palliative care

This is now being seen as an important and worthwhile part of care. Survey evidence shows that many later stage cancer patients suffer both from pain and other symptoms: there are already the skills and the drug therapies to ensue privacy, dignity and control in the last phase of life.

How we can achieve progress in cancer care?

Progress in cancer care now depends on using this new evidence base effectively to invest in the systems that will improve outcomes. How can middle income countries create the conditions in which a new generation of cancer professionals can "catch up"?

New infrastructures, roles and responsibilities

A major challenge facing those leading reform lies in creating new infrastructures and ultimately new roles and responsibilities within the context of Figure 9.1. In particular, much attention is now focussing upon the need to create and administratively support new working relationships between surgeons, radiotherapists and oncologists. In many cases, whilst these are evolving pragmatically in response to new patient demands and new treatment options, there is a danger that changes in both organisational behaviours and structures lag far behind what would be optimal in the light of technological progress. Figure 9.2 below highlights the parallel activities of these specialisms, which offer much scope for further development of more refined systems of networking and communication.

Improving the patients' experience: keeping up with the future

Two separate developments will determine the patients' experience of future cancer care. Increasing expectations by patients as consumers will lead health and social care services to become much more responsive to the individual, in the way that other service industries had started to become in the latter years of the 20th century. Coupled with this, targeted approaches to diagnosis and treatment will individualise care. People will have higher personal expectations, be less deferential to professionals and more willing to seek alternative care providers if dissatisfied. As a result, patients will be more involved in their care. They will take more responsibility for decisions rather than accepting a paternalistic "doctor knows best" approach. This will be fuelled partly by the Internet and competitive provider systems. In 20 years, the overwhelming majority of people in their 70s and 80s will be familiar with using the Internet to access information through the massive computing power that they will carry personally.

With patients having access to so much health information, they will need someone to interpret the huge volumes available, helping them assess the risks and benefits as well as determining what is relevant to them. These patient brokers will be compassionate but independent advocates who will act as patients' champions, guiding them through the system. They will be helped by intelligent algorithms to ensure patients understand screening and the

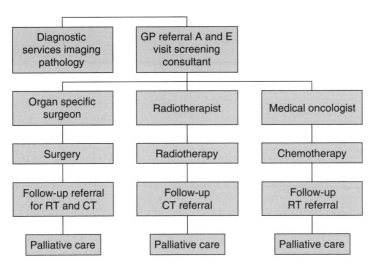

Figure 9.2   The cancer care pathway.

implications of early diagnosis. They will spell out what genetic susceptibility means and guide patients through the treatment options. Patients and health professionals will have confidence in computer-aided decision-making because they will have evidence that the programmes work.

However, cancer care will be a two-way street. Cancer patients will also coach doctors and other patients. With so many people expected to be living with cancer by 2020, they will have a great deal of knowledge and experience that professionals will need to tap into. Health professionals will be educated to accept that the person with cancer is an expert both about themselves and their illness. There will be continued interest in complementary medicines covering a wide range of talking, touching and pharmacological therapies operating outside the norms of conventional medical science. Improved regulation of practitioners in this area will enhance the quality of care provided and lead to better organisation of services.

How the service will be designed around patients' needs and expectations will be determined by the improved treatments available and their individualisation. Care in the early stages will be provided near to where patients live. Even the most sophisticated diagnostic machinery or robotic surgeon will be mobile, so much of this intervention will be carried out by technicians and nurses, with the most highly trained professionals in audio-visual contact from a distant base. When cancer centres developed mid 20th century, the diseases were relatively rare, and survival was low. Although distressing for patients when they were referred to a centre, their existence concentrated expertise. Cancer will be much more common, and as accepted as other chronic conditions, so that even when inpatient care is required, patients will be able to choose many places in the world where they will receive care at a "cancer hotel". But for many patients, even that option will not be necessary. Most new drugs will be given orally, so patients will be treated in their communities. However, this approach to cancer and other concomitant chronic conditions will place a huge burden on social services and families. Systems will be put in place to manage the on-going control of these diseases and conditions – psychologically as well as physically.

Improving treatment will increase focus on quality of life

Seventy per cent of the cancer budget is currently spent on care associated with the last 6 months of people's lives. Although many recognised that such treatment has more to do with the management of fear rather than the management of cancer, in the past, medical professionals had relatively few treatment options available and there has been limited awareness of which patients would benefit. There is also an institutional reluctance to destroy patients' hopes that has led to confusion between the limits of conventional medicines and reluctance to face the inevitable: by patients, their families and doctors. There is a widespread perception that if patients continue to be offered active anti-cancer treatment, there is the possibility that their health might be restored.

With better treatments, consumers of services (both patients and their carers) will be able to focus more on quality of life. Much of the fear associated with cancer will be mitigated. Demand for treatments with few side effects, or lower toxicity will be high, even if there are only quite modest survival gains. Yet, patients will only be treated who can benefit from the most expensive treatments and other approaches will be developed.

Creating incentives for investment and care quality

We can develop programmes to integrate cancer care into healthcare in the 21st century. The principal elements in the new model will be:

1. new kinds of partnership between patients and health professionals;
2. a stronger evidence base on care and treatment options, which will be accessible through web sites to local professionals;
3. a shift from emphasis on items of hardware towards software systems;
4. new informatics for measuring quality and clinical governance;

5. greater emphasis on networking and teamwork;
6. a commitment to learning and adaptation through national and international links;
7. a shift away from inpatient care toward ambulatory care;
8. targeting of patients at high risk for genetic reasons;
9. targeting of disease prevention and treatment in socially deprived areas;
10. a strategic role for health funds with use of managed care systems.

In the past, many nations have demonstrated great strength in their extraordinary trust in doctors and other health professionals to give good care, even with limited resources. The aim of the programme would be to ensure that such qualities could continue to thrive in a changing health environment. This should be regarded as essential for international competitiveness and accreditation.

The programme would cover initiatives in the following six areas, and for each one, we define the first steps that could produce real results in 2–3 years.

Prevention

Here, the critical policy is to strengthen programmes for tobacco control. The WHO programme sets the framework, but any general reductions in smoking will take time both to take place and to impact on health status. Given the urgency of the problem there may well be a case for special measures to reach high-risk groups such as men over 30 who have been smokers for 10 years or more, women during pregnancy, patients with diabetes or CHD who are already being treated (Figure 9.3).

Screening and early detection

A start has to be made here in the two key areas of mammography and screening for cancer of the cervix. It is essential to move forward to ensure population coverage on a 3-year basis. Screening for colo-rectal cancer could begin through pilot schemes in high-risk areas.

Diagnostics and assessment

Clearer standards need to be set for speed of treatment and increasing information on available options for treatment. The main challenge will be to improve staging so that more patients will be treated quickly at earlier stages.

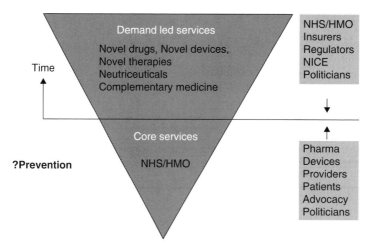

Figure 9.3   The cancer demand pyramid.

Treatment and care

There will be a move towards more complex choices with differing sequences and options for surgery/chemotherapy/radiotherapy. Therapy will be longer and more intense with greater urgency about monitoring the patient's experience and fatigue.

Follow up and continuing treatment

It will be vital to improve medical records to ensure that patients at risk are recalled. This will be particularly important with longer-term prophylaxis for breast cancer.

Palliative care

There has been some progress towards improving the service in palliative care. For example, in Hungary patients' experience of cancer has been improved through the initiative of the Soros Foundation, but much more needs to be done. We would strongly recommend a one-off investment programme to assist with the transition. For middle-income countries there could be international/charitable sponsorship for National Fight Cancer Funds (e.g. $50 m each for Hungary and the Czech Republic, and $100 m for Poland). A strategy

group with representatives from national Ministries, Health Funds, oncologists and patient groups is required. This would set directions and the full
time Fight Cancer Fund Manager would report to this.

Funding of key investments

Throughout this text we have frequently drawn attention to the formidable
nature of the challenge involved in making good choices for long-term
investment of limited funds. Whilst we do not wish to engage here in a
debate regarding the well-known arguments on the respective economic
and social merits of private versus public funding mechanisms, it would be
naïve not to recognise the reality: that in addition to the established state or
national social insurance fund financing systems, there is ample anecdotal
evidence of a flourishing private sector approach based largely upon out of
pocket payments by those who can afford it. Whilst the funding of cancer
services is unquestionably a high priority for public systems, the scale of
growth in demand, fuelled both by patient numbers and new technology
options, could well see a further expansion of private funding, with all the
well-known attendant stresses associated with inequity of access based upon
a broader experience of this dynamic, clearly indicates that difficult, far
more publicly transparent decisions, will have to be made as to what core
services can be provide by public systems and which, albeit reluctantly,
access will be limited or delayed.

The need for national cancer plans

As illustrated in Figure 9.4, the social insurance funds and national ministries
in many countries face a massive challenge in formulating long-term strategies for allocating limited funds to a range of services. Many face uncertain
futures, in terms of income streams, which are heavily dependent upon
national economic performance. There are many other competing priorities
besides cancer, and above all, the need to push through funding and organisational reforms on a grand scale. Somehow within this context, the concept
of a national cancer investment plan, supported by the relevant professional
bodies, needs to be established with a clearer set of investment and funding
priorities, which are compatible with the wider reform programme.

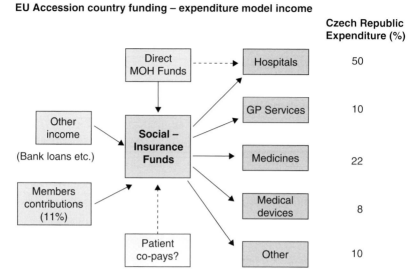

Figure 9.4   Funding mechanisms and investment priorities.

We would suggest that the following components should be high priorities in this plan:

1. stronger management capability in key local centres especially in areas of systems design and utilisation;
2. expansion of screening programmes and management to ensure population coverage;
3. encouraging 'pluralism' through private/public partnership;
4. design new informatics or quality measurement and for networking among professionals;
5. training of doctors and health professionals in new skills;
6. design of protocols and care pathways;
7. investing in new management and upgrading of diagnostic/treatment systems so as to ensure most effective use;
8. developing international links and increasing research/clinical trial participation;
9. organising workshops and conferences to increase international co-operation in improving cancer services.

The Fight Cancer Funds would increase confidence in change and the momentum towards service improvement. They would be essential to ensuring that the health professions in the NMS can play their full role. In the interwar period, cancer services were beginning to develop strongly, for example through the Marie Curie Institute in Warsaw and the Masaryk Institute in Brno. European Union membership gives an opportunity for a move towards international collaboration and even leadership in reducing the social and human costs of cancer.

Key conclusions and recommendations

We set these in the specific context of the new member States of the EU, but we would see the model as being of relevance to a wide range both of developed and of middle-income countries. The NMS face challenges in reducing the disease burden from cancer. It is already much higher than in the old EU and is set to rise further without effective action. Levels of expenditure on cancer services, mainly for treatment, are currently low at 3–5% of total health expenditures. Survival outcomes achieved in the 1990s were about two-thirds of those in Western Europe. This was a remarkable achievement given the low level of resources available for treating patients diagnosed in 1990–1994.

Without modernisation the core strength of commitment from dedicated clinicians is likely to be eroded as some younger professionals migrate. There will be problems in meeting new and challenging standards for clinical governance. There is a new model of cancer care, which leads towards balanced and co-ordinated investment in prevention, screening and treatment and follow-up care. The model also supplies many opportunities or international partnership, where greater participation in clinical trials has already been a good start.

Use of this model is essential to achieving reductions in cancer incidence and mortality. We are impressed by the potential for services in the NMS to catch up, but the opportunities must be taken soon.

Recommendations

We recommend:

- The creation of National Cancer Strategies, which will focus investment and service development. These can set out coherent programmes for prevention, screening and treatment and follow-up care. Key targets and timelines will back these up and resource plans for staff, equipment and drug budgets. The plans will be based on partnership between

Governments, Insurance Funds, health professionals and patient groups. Furthermore, we encourage developing and attracting funding sources for the Fight Cancer Funds, which will give a start to the strategies. The new model of cancer care requires a one-time investment in care programmes, staffing and Institute of Cancer Therapeutic (ICT). It is hardly realistic to expect that the investment required can be found from existing health funds during a time of great pressure on public sector budgets. Possible contributors to the Funds would be the EU, The World bank, philanthropists such as the Soros Foundation, and corporate donors.

- The development of national training/staffing programmes to secure the range of new skills required for the plan opening up skill development both for newer recruits and for experienced staff working in the service.
- The development of a key leader programme for staff in their 30s including short-term international placements and opportunities for leadership training.
- The creation of a national initiative in quality assurance, which would collaborate with major centres in developing networks and protocols. This is crucial for using the full potential and commitment of staff in the services.
- The development of roles and opportunities for specialist nurses who can make a crucial contribution to screening, treatment and follow-up care.
- Further development of a national initiative in palliative and terminal care. Many patients are suffering from both tremendous pain and distress from other symptoms. The aims of privacy, dignity and control in the last phases of life are vital and achievable.

For example in New Europe EU Accession is already having unexpected and positive effects in economic terms. It could also be the opportunity for new social initiatives. We present here a programme of investment, which could allow "catching-up" in process quality and outcomes. There can be new partnership to reduce disease burdens and to add substantial life expectancy.

Increased investment

The investment programme would cover: prevention, the extension of screening, the development of information technology, the reorganisation of services into ambulatory care centres, staff training, skill development, and follow up and palliative care. For a country of 20 m people, an initial investment of $100–200 m would be required, followed by an expenditure of

$50 m over 5 years for continuing and progressive re-engineering of service. Assuming 100,000 new patients a year this would imply a rise in cost per patient on average of $2500 over 5 years. Such a rise in spending may well come about anyway through cost pressures and extended use of new therapies: we are suggesting that it should be targeted to the new staged programme. This programme does not achieve results through heavy spending on new and specialised buildings and equipment. In fact, much of the IT can be taken from that already in use. Some of the investment could be funded by reducing spending on hospital admissions, and some of the staffing can be funded through offering new career opportunities to staff already working in cancer services. The programme depends above all on the drive, leadership and can do capability of the small band of men and women who make cancer services in each country. New kinds of private and non-profit enterprises can play crucial roles.

The developing world

The global incidence of cancer is dramatically increasing due to rapidly ageing populations in most countries. By the year 2020, there will be 20 million new cancer patients each year. Seventy per cent of them will live in countries that between them will have less than 5% of the resources for cancer control. We have seen an explosion in our understanding of the disease at a molecular level and are now poised to see remarkable advances in prevention, screening and treatment.

Dramatic technological change is likely in surgery, radiotherapy and chemotherapy leading to increased cure rates.[1] The completion of the human genome project will almost certainly bring sophisticated genetic risk assessment methods requiring careful integration into existing screening programmes.[2] Preventive strategies could considerably reduce the global disease burden at low cost. And, palliative care to relieve pain and suffering should be a basic right of all cancer patients. The next 25 years will be a time of unprecedented change in the way in which we will control cancer. However, the optimal organisation of prevention and detection programmes, as well as treatment services, are universal problems in all economic environments.

The world is in a health transition. Infection as a major cause of suffering and death is giving way to new epidemics of non-communicable disorders such as cardiovascular disease, diabetes and cancer.[3] Different countries are in different stages of this evolution depending on their age, structure and economy. Some countries are faced with a double burden with increasing infection problems compounded by surging cancer rates. This is fuelled in part by the globalisation of unhealthy lifestyles.[4]

The original WHO Cancer Unit started in Geneva in 1961. Over the last decade it concentrated mainly on the provision of palliative care facilities becoming the Cancer and Palliative Care Unit. The Cancer Programme was housed in the International Agency for Research on Cancer in Lyon.[5] This research institute is funded by 18 countries to carry out research into the epidemiology and causes of cancer. The mission of the current Cancer Programme is to reduce the incidence, morbidity and mortality of cancer in each of the 191 countries belonging to the United Nations. It has now been integrated into the non-communicable disease division of the WHO in Geneva.

To achieve this objective it is necessary to provide advice on the best standard of detection, screening and care possible in very different economic environments. Practice guidelines are an essential tool from primary through to tertiary care in ensuring quality, equity and consistency in health service provision. They also serve as a vital tool for developing a financially sustainable service and auditing the quality of care provided.[6,7,8]

Guidelines for prevention

The instigation of comprehensive national cancer control programmes has been an essential component in WHO's work.[9] Unfortunately, their success depends on finding local enthusiasm, expertise and political will, which need to continue for long periods of time. The incubation period for cancer far exceeds the voting cycle of democratically elected governments. This makes politicians favour more immediately visible strategies to deal with cancer such as screening or the construction of cancer centres. It is estimated that 30% of the current 10 million new cancers are due to tobacco use, 30% due to dietary factors and 15% due to infection. Other possible causes attract disproportionate media attention and thus public awareness includes: electromagnetic field, radiation from power lines and cell phones, stress and alcohol. Several attempts have been made to produce guidelines for cancer prevention and to set realistic long-term targets.[10,11,12] A major problem is the absolute requirement for multi-agency working between those involved in education, health care and social services. Few of such guidelines have ever met their targets, essentially because of "cancer fatigue" leading to poor compliance by the population.

Tobacco

Optimal use of current knowledge could reduce the overall cancer incidence by at least 3 million. We need to look for long-term solutions here. The politics of tobacco is a complex conspiratorial web of industrialists, farmers, manufacturers, politicians and the pensions business all looking after their own interests.[13] Governments are naturally cautious of reducing cigarette consumption in many countries as the economy simply collapses. In democracies, they are subject to intense lobbying. In less democratic societies corruption, using the massive profits generated by the industry, usually achieves the desired end point. Advertising blatantly exploits the young of the developing world, associating images of sex, success and wealth with cigarettes as a lifestyle marker. The solutions are complex and require considerable political will, but with forceful and concerted international action against cigarette promotion we could reduce cancer incidence by 20% by the year 2020. The WHO is developing an international framework convention to bring about a cohesive legal strategy to reduce tobacco use.[14]

Diet

Dietary modification could result in a further 30% reduction across the board.[15] The problem is refining the educational message and getting it right in different communities. Changing our current high fat, low fibre diet (with a low fruit and vegetable intake) are common themes for cancer prevention. But many features of the modern western diet are now being adapted globally as branded fast food makers seek out new markets. Again, political will is necessary to reduce the costs to the public of healthy foods. We need to get more data so that we can make firmer recommendations. The European Prospective Investigation into Diet and Cancer (EPIC) study currently in progress is a good example where painstaking data and serum collection on 400,000 Europeans could, over the years, provide a vast resource for investigating prospectively the complex interrelationships between diet and cancer.[16] Cancer incidence varies enormously across Europe providing an excellent natural laboratory for such studies.

Moreover, interventional epidemiology, using rigorous controlled studies, could produce the evidence that could lead to major changes. The current problem is the difficulty in making dietary advice specific and in some countries affordable. Although several groups have produced guidelines, there is so far little data about their uptake or significance in large populations. Clearly, more refined messages are going to be necessary if dietary interventions are really going to make a dent on cancer statistics.

Infection

Infection causes around 15% of cancer worldwide and is potentially preventable. This proportion is greater in the developing world where an estimated 22% of cancer has an infectious cause.[17] Hepatitis B immunisation in children has significantly reduced the incidence of infection in China, Korea and West Africa. Shortly, we will see if it has reduced the incidence of hepatoma, which begins in endemic regions by the third decade of life. The unconfirmed trends are already encouraging.[18] Cancer of the cervix, the commonest women's cancer in parts of India and Latin America, is clearly associated with certain subtypes of human papilloma virus. Vaccines are now becoming available and entering trial.[19] Helicobacter pylori is associated with stomach cancer. Here, without any intervention, there has been a remarkable downward trend in incidence worldwide. Dissecting out the complex factors involved including food storage, contamination, preparation and content is a considerable challenge. Other cancer causing infections are Schistosomiasis, the liver fluke, the human T cell leukaemia virus and the ubiquitous HIV. Although geographically localised, their prevention by lifestyle changes and vaccination programmes are realistic short-term goals. Clearly, the effectiveness of any infection control or immunisation programme at reducing the cancer burden will depend on many factors and require careful research, field evaluation and economic analysis before individual guidelines can be constructed.

Cancer detection

Screening in many countries is also an important tool. Careful targeting is required – breast cancer is simply not a major problem in many parts of the world. Again, the cost of the technology required must match the gain. Low cost direct inspection techniques for oral and cervical cancer by health workers seem attractive to achieve tumour down staging and hence better

survival results.[20,21] Unfortunately, the evaluation of cervicoscopy programmes in India and China have shown surprisingly poor results in terms
of overall effectiveness.[22] It remains to be seen whether intra-vital staining
using acetic acid can enhance specificity with little cost. A major cost in
instituting any screening procedure is simply getting the message to the people and then developing the logistics, often under difficult conditions.
Cultural barriers may be insurmountable without better education, especially of girls, who as mothers will become responsible for family health.
Low technology tests have low specificity so flooding already hard pressed
secondary care facilities with patients with non-life threatening abnormalities. Detailed field assessment preferably in a randomised setting is essential
before firm recommendations can be made.

Treatment guidelines

There is good evidence that patients with potentially curable cancers such as
Hodgkin's Disease, childhood leukaemia, Burkitt's lymphoma and testicular
cancer fare less well in poorer countries. Getting good results here has to be the
priority. Adjuvant therapy is of proven value in breast and colon cancer and yet
rarely given in many parts of the world. Guidelines for referral, treatment and
care are urgently needed. Effective facilities for the safe administration of
radiotherapy and chemotherapy are essential everywhere. Such guidelines
must be locally adapted and be matched by the appropriate expertise.

The WHO has produced recommendations on the essential drugs
required for cancer therapy.[23,24] Over the last 5 years, several new anti-
cancer drugs have been aggressively marketed. Most of these are costly and
produce only limited benefits. We have divided currently available anti-cancer
drugs into three priority groups: curable cancers and those cancers where
the cost-benefit ratio clearly favours drug treatment can be managed appro-
priately with regimens based on only 17 drugs. All of these are available,
at relatively low cost, as generic preparations. The wide availability of these
drugs should be the first priority. A second group of drugs may have some
advantages in certain clinical situations. Based on current evidence, drugs in
the third group are judged as currently not essential for the effective delivery of
cancer care. Adequate supportive care programmes with the widespread availability of effective drugs for pain control are of considerably greater importance. The adoption of these priorities will help to optimise the effectiveness

and efficiency of chemotherapy and ensure equitable access to essential drugs especially in low resource environments.

Psychosocial care

All cancer patients require good psychosocial and palliative care within the context of their own culture. Health professionals now convey far more information to patients about cancer. This needs to be backed up by careful counselling of patient and carers. Empowering all health professionals, carers and those administering health systems is an essential part. Complementary therapies can improve the quality of life and put patients back in control. Nurses here have made dramatic strides in tackling the complex interfaces of palliative care. This needs to be exported to areas where nurses are still regarded as doctors' handmaidens. Pain control is a vital part of cancer management and yet there are still many places in which morphine is unavailable for legal reasons. Ironically, these countries are often the main sources of illicit opium derived products. Education, information and political persuasion are the key to the future. Simple process guidelines such as the WHO cancer pain ladder have been remarkably successful in conveying a simple message to those involved in cancer patient care.[25]

The WHO cancer priority ladder

A series of 12 pilot projects are being set up with Health Ministries around the world. The epidemiological and economic spectra of the pilot settings differs considerably. A consortium of international agencies, unilateral aid providers, educational organisations, professional bodies, charities and the healthcare industry is being put together. The aim is to offer a comprehensive programme of expertise channelled through the Health Departments but with the full involvement of professionals already involved in cancer care.[26] It is vital that this process encourages rather than stifles local enthusiasm and innovation.

The central plank of this initiative will be the WHO cancer priority ladder. This provides internationally agreed priorities for developing effective cancer control. It needs to be carefully adapted to local circumstance. Tobacco control is a ubiquitous problem but the methods used to achieve long-term control will differ. Furthermore, careful political consideration across a range of government departments will be necessary especially in those countries where tobacco is a major source of employment and taxation. Infection control is an achievable target but is geographically very specific. Hepatitis B, for example, is fortunately rare in many developing countries and so universal vaccination strategies to reduce the incidence of hepatoma would be inappropriate. Encouraging healthy eating and discouraging food manufacturing practices that increase fat and lower fibre content is a cheap intervention that will reduce the burden of cardiovascular disease as well as cancer.

A curable cancer programme is essential as a tool for political persuasion. By looking at cancer positively people can be convinced to take action. Many in the past have been critical of the large sums spent on cancer patients by tertiary care facilities in many poorer countries. But the effective organisation of services into a hub-and-spoke model similar to that currently being enacted in the UK[27] could focus care where it can be most effective. Ensuring the availability of basic cancer surgery, radiotherapy and chemotherapy for potentially curable cancers provides the first step in setting up a comprehensive cancer service. Agreed referral and clinical care guidelines which can subsequently be audited are an essential component. Furthermore, this provides a cadre of interested professionals who can be encouraged to take a more holistic view of the cancer problem in their country. This may be enhanced by visiting review programmes such as the WHO Cancer Advisory Programme. This scheme, piloted in Morocco and Vietnam, provides site visits over 3 years by a group of experienced oncologists and epidemiologists. This allows leaders of the local oncology community to review in an informal setting their future plans as well as make personal international contacts. As well as reviewing cancer treatment capability, such programmes encourage the local ownership of comprehensive cancer control, from prevention through to palliative care by those involved in resource allocation. Cancer registries can cost less than £7000 ($10,000) per year to run and can provide an excellent database for time trends and measuring the impact of specific initiatives.

Private sector involvement

These developments must also embrace the private sector. Increasingly the emergent middle class in poorer economies are turning to the private sector for healthcare. If specialist services are not available then there is no choice but to travel abroad often at considerable expense especially when compared to average earnings in many countries. Encouraging private sector involvement locally not only makes economic sense for future consumers but also provides for a technological trickle down effect.

Developing programmes to ensure the earlier detection of cancer is also important. These range from educational initiatives through to formal population based screening strategies. In many economic environments mammography and cervical cytology may be inappropriate interventions because of their cost. However, there are several potential interventions that can result in tumour down staging and these need to be prioritised.

Specialist nurse education is a further priority. A major problem is the considerable variation in level of education expected and achieved in many countries. Utilising all professional skills to their best advantage must take precedence over turf wars. The use of nurses in chemotherapy delivery areas and radiographers in the delivery of radiotherapy can be enhanced by introducing basic clinical decision-making skills following present guidelines. Psychosocial and information needs are best handled by those working closest to the patient and their family. Developing the role of the nurse must be a high priority in most settings.

Evaluation, audit, education and clinical research are all interrelated. Good research can be done anywhere provided the problem addressed is carefully chosen. Unfortunately, there is a great tendency for physicians in developing countries to wish to emulate colleagues in the developed world. In doing so, unrealistic high technology projects are attempted, which are doomed unless part of a pre-agreed international programme. Realistic assessment of research strategies with proper peer review is essential.

Platform technology programmes are the beginning of international aid. Once a successful National Cancer Programme is established many of its features can be adapted to neighbouring countries with similar characteristics. The WHO will continue to encourage this type of development alongside traditional methods of aid.

Conclusion

The construction of guidelines, properly adapted to the circumstances of the developing world, provides a useful tool to improve the quality of global cancer care. Such guidelines can consider common clinical problems in most malignant disease and be tailored to local circumstances. They form part of the prioritisation strategy recommended by WHO in the implementation of National Cancer Programmes. Prevention, detection, treatment and psychosocial care can all be covered utilising local facilities and referral networks. Guidelines have considerable educational value in the training of a wide range of health professionals in cancer management. Above all they encourage the delivery of cancer care in the most efficient and cost effective way possible.

REFERENCES

1. Imperial Cancer Research Fund (1995) *A Vision for Cancer*. London.
2. Holtzman N.A. and Shapiro D. (1998) Genetic testing and public policy. *British Medical Journal* 316: 852–856.
3. WHO (1998) *The World Health Report*. WHO, Geneva.
4. Murray C.J. and Lopez A.D. (1996) *The Global Burden of Disease*. Harvard University Press, Boston.
5. International Agency for Research on Cancer (1997) *Biennial Report*. IARC Press, Lyon.
6. Parkin D., Whelan S., Ferlay J., Raymond L. and Young J. (1997) *Cancer in Five Continents. Vol. VII.* IARC Scientific Publications, Lyon.
7. IARC/WHO (1998) *Cancer in Five Continents. Electronic Database for Cancer.* IARC/WHO, Lyon.
8. Murray C.J. and Lopez A.D. (1997) Regional patterns of disability free life expectancy and disability adjusted life expectancy. *Lancet* 349: 1347–1352.
9. Sikora K. (1999) Developing a global strategy for cancer. *European Journal of Cancer* 35: 24–31.
10. Austoker J. (1995) *Cancer Prevention in Primary Care*. BMJ Books, London.
11. Department of Health (1993) *The Health of the Nation*. UK Department of Health, UK.
12. Stationery Office (1998) *Our Healthier Nation*. Stationery Office, London.
13. Taylor P. (1984) *Smoke Ring – The Politics of Tobacco*. Bodley Head, London.
14. Yach D. (1999) *An International Framework Convention for Tobacco Control*. WHO Publications, Geneva.
15. Doll R. and Peto R. (1985) *The Causes of Cancer*. Oxford University Press, Oxford.
16. Riboli E. and Kaaks R. (1997) European perspective investigation into cancer and nutrition. *International Journal of Epidemiology* 26(Suppl. 1): 6–14.
17. Pisani P., Parkin D.M., Munoz N. and Ferlay J. (1997) Cancer and infection: estimates of the attributable fraction in 1990. *Cancer Epidemiology, Biomarkers and Prevention* 6: 387–400.
18. Jack A.D. (1998) Follow up of the vaccinated cohort. Hepatitis B immunization and prevention of cirrhosis and hepatocellular carcinoma in Sub-Saharan Africa: Banjul.

19. Monsonego J. and Franco E. (1996) *Cervical Cancer Control. General Statements and Guidelines.* EUROGIN, Paris.
20. Nene B.M., Deshpande S., Jayant K. et al. (1996) Early detection of cervical cancer by visual inspection. *International Journal of Cancer* 68: 770–773.
21. Sankaranarayanan R. (1997) Health care auxilliaries in the detection and prevention of oral cancer. *European Journal of Cancer* 33: 149–154.
22. Sankaranarayanan R., Syamalakumai B., Wesley R. et al. (1997) Visual inspection as a screening test for cervical cancer control in developing countries. In: *New Developments in Cervical Cancer Screening and Prevention* (eds Franco and Monsonego). Paris, pp. 411–421.
23. Sikora K., Advani S., Korolthouck V. et al. (1999) Essential drugs for cancer therapy: a WHO consultation. *Annuals of Oncology* 10: 1–6.
24. World Health Organisation (1994) Essential drugs for cancer chemotherapy. *Bulletin of the World Health Organisation* 72: 693–698.
25. WHO (1998) *Cancer Pain Relief.* WHO, Geneva.
26. WHO (1995) *National Cancer Control Programmes.* Policies and managerial guidelines. WHO, Geneva.
27. Department of Health (1995) *Recommendations for Commissioning Cancer Services. Report of the Expert Advisory Group on Cancer.* Department of Health, London.

10

Cancer's economic impact on society

We will never have enough money to do everything

The picture painted of cancer care in 2025 is one where cancer is incidental to day-to-day living. Cancers will not necessarily be eradicated but that will not cause patients the anxiety that it would in 2003. People will have far greater control over their medical destinies than in 2003. Compared with 2003, there is little doubt that patients in all socio-economic groups will be better informed. In addition, surgery and chemotherapy will not be rationed on grounds of age since all interventions will be less damaging – psychologically as well as physically.

How true this picture will be will depend on whether the technological advances – outlined in previous sections – will emerge. Will people, for example, really live in "smart" houses where their televisions play a critical role in monitoring their health and well-being. It is also dependent on health-care professionals working alongside each other, valuing the input of carers who, even more than in 2003, will provide voluntary support because of the number of people in older age groups compared with those of working age.

The reality for cancer care may be rather different. The ideal will exist for a minority of patients, but the majority may not have access to the full range of services. Old people in 2025, having been relatively poor all their lives, may suffer from cancer and a huge range of co-morbidities that will limit their quality of life. Looking after them all – rich and poor – will place great strains on younger people: will there be enough of them to provide the care? As with all health issues the question of access will be determined by cost and political will. In 2003, a cancer patient consumed about £20,000 worth of direct medical care costs (70% spent in the last 6 months of life) not including the costs of addressing other medical and social problems. Conservatively, with patients living with cancer, rather than dying from it, and with access to new technologies this could be £100,000 per patient per year by 2025. In theory, cancer care could absorb an ever-increasing proportion of the health-care budget. Will this be a reflection of what patients want? Probably "yes". Patients' surveys in 2003 revealed that three quarters of the population believed that cancer care should be the National Health Service (NHS) priority with no other disease area being even a close second.

But to achieve that expenditure – and assuming that part of the health service will be funded from taxation – the tax rate might have to rise to 60%. Inevitably, there will be conflicting demands on resources: the choice may be drugs or care costs. And how are the costs computed? There are many angles to consider. One line of argument is that in 2025, although the technology will be expensive, it will be used more judiciously than it could be in 2003, since it will be better targeted. Another argument suggests that when patients are empowered they use less and fewer expensive medicines, in effect lowering the overall costs. An extension of that argument is that although costs will increase for treating each individual patient, the overall costs will decrease because when patients do have to be treated as inpatients – be it in a hospital or cancer hotel – the length of stay will be shorter, treatment will be minimally invasive and there will be less morbidity and cost associated with the intervention.

However, by concentrating more effort into a shorter treatment time, access to services will be greater and each bed will have a higher patient turnover (partly driven by the success of new treatments, so more people will demand them). Costs per treatment rise, and, because people live longer lifetime costs of cancer care rise along with co-morbidity costs. Politicians will be faced with a real dilemma: if the population of cancer sufferers stays stable or increases, the cost of keeping them alive will be greater than the cost of educating the next generation. Will cancer care need to be rationed in a draconian way? Other considerations that may have financial implications include the impact on voluntary organisations: if cancer loses its capacity to frighten patients what will that do to the fund-raising abilities of cancer research and cancer care charities?

One other development in 2025 will be the political power of old people. Not only will more of them be living longer than in 2003, their chronic problems will not necessarily incapacitate them physically or mentally. The educated gerontocracy will have high expectations that will have been sharpened through the first two decades of the 21st century and they will not tolerate the standards of care offered to many old people in 2003. They will wield considerable influence.

Will a tax-based health system be able to fund their expectations? Politicians will have to consider the alignment between patients' requirements, and taxpayers' and voters' wishes. Fewer than 50% of voters paid tax in 2003, and the percentage of tax-paying voters is set to fall as the population ages. Will the younger taxpayers of 2025 tolerate the selfish wishes of non-taxpayers? The interests of voters may be very different to the interests of taxpayers. It seems likely, therefore, that the days of an exclusively tax-funded health service are numbered. Co-payments and deductibles will be the new vocabulary of health-care finance.

Future governments may be forced to provide a core package of care for the whole population. Individuals would be expected to top-up their health fund through insurance and there could be systems in place that delegates responsibility of health-care funding to local decision-makers – effectively putting patients in control of funds. Some people may find that high-cost interventions may be not available to them. Will the new generation of chemotherapeutic agents be so prohibitively expensive that treatment once more focuses on the traditional approaches surgery and radiotherapy? Patients, however, could be offered financial incentives to live as healthy a life as possible – with greater choice comes greater responsibility.

Whatever system is put in place there is the prospect of a major socioeconomic division in 2025. A small percentage of the elderly population will have made suitable provision for their retirement, both in terms of health and welfare, but the vast majority will not be properly prepared. Policymakers need to start planning now as they are doing for the looming pensions crisis. The most productive way forward may be to start to involve cancer patient and health advocacy groups in the debate, to ensure that difficult decisions are reached by consensus.

Societal change will create new challenges in the provision of care. A decline in hierarchical religious structures, a reduction in family integrity through increasing divorce, greater international mobility and the increased selfishness of a consumer driven culture will leave many lonely and with no psychological crutch to lean on at the onset of serious illness. There will be a global shortage of carers – the unskilled, low paid but essential component of any health delivery system. The richer parts of the world are now harnessing this from the poorer countries but eventually the supply of this precious human capital will evaporate.

New financial structures will emerge with novel consortia from the pharmaceutical, financial and health-care sectors enabling people to buy into the level of care they wish to pay for. Cancer, cardiovascular disease and dementia will be controlled and join today's list of chronic diseases, such as diabetes, asthma and hypertension. Hospitals will become attractive health hotels run by competing private sector providers. Global franchises will provide speciality therapies through these structures similar to the internationally branded shops in today's malls. Governments will have long ceased to deliver care. Britain's NHS, one of the last centralised systems to disappear, will convert to UK Health – a regulator and safety net insurer by 2012.

The ability of technology to improve health is assured. But this will come at a price – the direct costs of providing it and the care costs of the increasingly elderly population it will produce. We will simply run out of things to die from. New ethical and moral dilemmas will arise as we seek the holy grail of compressed morbidity. Living long and dying fast will become the mantra of 21st century medicine. Our cancer future will emerge from the interaction of four factors: the success of new technology, society's willingness to pay, future healthcare delivery systems and the financial mechanisms that underpin them.

11

Improving the patient experience

The cancer treatment services have been developed for short episodes of treatment and have been distinguished by intensive professional direction: now they have to adapt to a new situation when they will need to offer more information on options and continuing support. New approaches are needed and a new commitment in order to improve the quality of life of survivors. In the past, cancer patients have complained more than others about lack of information during treatment. Survivors have been found to have a significantly poorer quality of life compared to their peers. Data for the US show the following:

- The number of cancer survivors rose from 3 to 10 million from 1971 to 2001.
- 64% of adults whose cancer is diagnosed today can expect to be living in 5-year time.
- Breast cancer survivors make up the largest group of cancer survivors (22%) followed by prostate cancer survivors (17%) and colo-rectal cancer survivors (11%).
- The majority (61%) of cancer survivors are aged 65 or older.
- An estimated one out of every six people aged over 65 is a cancer survivor.[1]

This increase in prevalence in certain cancers will result in significant changes for patients who will experience living with cancer as a chronic disease for many years or even decades, not just days or months. Patients will be concerned about the impact of treatment on quality of life in the short term and on their ability to function in the longer term. Younger patients will fear loss of income and problems of employment. They will have to deal with the social and economic effects of cancer treatment as well as the physical side-effects of the disease and its treatment. Cancer services will have to develop in a number of different dimensions. These will include:

1. Communication with patients and carers on treatment choices.
2. Increasing the role of primary care in providing support for cancer patients as well as in early identification and diagnosis.
3. Developing choice in location and timing of treatment.
4. Improving cancer rehabilitation and longer-term support.
5. Improving access to complementary therapies.
6. Improving palliative care and end of life support.

Improving communication

Patients often express frustration at the brevity of information they receive on cancer. The President's Cancer Panel recently convened a meeting with European cancer survivors:

Speakers, particularly those who were longer-term survivors, noted that when they were diagnosed, they were given little or no information about their disease. Further there were no readily available information resources, and no internet, now often the most relied upon information source by both newly diagnosed and longer-term survivors.[2]

Some of the testimony from European patients showed just far there is to go:

I was always … looking for his right ward, for the room in which to undergo the CAT scan … for scintigraphy, for X-rays, bronchoscopy, etcetera. And all of this without synergy, and often, I myself had to explain to the doctor on duty what was wrong with me … everything is in my hands, my fight against cancer, my fight against the treatment by the medical professionals, and lastly, my fight against the system of how patients are followed up.[3]

It is so easy to do it differently: an open attitude to questions, interest in your personal situation, a telephone number to call in case of panic. These are really experiences that help.[4]

Improving the patient experience

A few simple changes could make a difference for most cancer patients in helping them through the patient journey. There are also some specific treatments where it may be vitally important to give patients much more information. Five-year follow-up of patients with prostate cancer has shown that people who are treated by surgery are much more likely to have serious problems with incontinence and impotence than patients treated with radio-therapy. In the UK, the number of trans-urethral resection of the prostrate (TURPS) operations has in fact halved since there was more awareness of these effects. It is now part of good professional practice, even minimum clinical governance, to ensure that patients are informed about the risks and benefits of a particular treatment.

A patient in the UK diagnosed with colo-rectal cancer in 2002 set out his views on how communication could be improved:

Primarily I would have liked the initial phase to have been more rapid! Waiting 6 months for a diagnosis was not really acceptable and it seems amazing that the ulcer was not seen with the rigid proctoscope. Another doctor I spoke to suggested that I was lucky that it didn't take a year. I was only seen at the hospital when I was because I kept pushing. Once everything was underway, I have no complaints about my treatment, though the thought that I would not have had oxaliplatin other than being part of the EXPERT trial is very frightening!

I would have liked a formal mechanism to obtain copies of all tests, scans, etc. at every stage. Some of these I obtained, but this was only on the basis of asking and hoping that someone did something about it. The colo-rectal specialist nurse and research nurse were very good at organising this early on but it hasn't been maintained.[5]

Among the most powerful accounts of poor communication and denial of access to treatment was another Report from the President Panel "Voices of a broken system." Even well informed patients in the US report great problems about access to care.

When you are fighting for your life which I was, it is virtually more than you can do to also fight the system every inch of the way ... I also want to point out that I am a middle class person. I have supportive family. I have an incredible network of friends. I'm also about to serve in my 11th year in the legislature, so I have skills, and knowledge, and at least perceived power and perceived access to the press that many people don't have. Yet despite all of that I had an incredible struggle to get all I needed for myself.[6]

There is also some survey evidence showing more positive developments. One survey of long-term survivors of lung cancer showed that 50% said that cancer had helped them to view their lives more positively and 71% described themselves as hopeful about the future.[7] Even so, 22% of respondents had distressed mood and scored low on depression scales. A study of long-term survivors of breast cancer (average of 6.3 years earlier) also showed that quality of life was good.

This was a large group of women, and the good news is that we could find very little wrong with the emotional or physical health of most of them.[8]

Increasing patient information

For patients at the treatment stage there is now strong evidence from many countries that patients want more information.

Many studies have suggested that patients with cancer believe they are not given enough information. Cassileh and colleagues found that most cancer patients in the USA wanted detailed information about their cancer whether the news was good or bad. This finding has been confirmed in surveys of patients with cancer in the UK, North America and Australia. A large study in the UK, involving 2231 patients, found that 87% of participants preferred to have as much information as possible: good or bad.[9]

There are a number of simple ways in which communication could be improved. Mills and Sullivan listed six functions of information for patients: to gain control; to reduce anxiety; to improve compliance; to create realistic expectations; to promote self-care and participation; and to generate feelings of safety and security.[10]

The key step here is to start and build on e-mail communication so that each patient can have a care programme. A recent survey of breast surgeons in the UK showed that currently they are making virtually no use of the internet. In fact, there was far less use than in many more mundane areas of life.[11]

E-mail communication can give a list of useful web sites for patient support group and information on treatment. It could give a contact point for patients with queries in the event of emergency. We see such a service as being well within the reach of most large centres, and it could make a great contribution to improving the patient experience.

Developing the role of primary care

In systems and countries with primary care, gate keeping the role of primary care in cancer services is bound to expand from initial referral through to palliative care. The accuracy of referral affects the speed of diagnosis and staging. Family doctors will often be asked for advice on therapies. They will have to manage longer-term support programmes and they will have the main role in shared care. In the UK, the original Calman–Hine report stressed that the role of the General Practitioner (GP) was central, yet little seems to have happened to follow this up effectively. A report by the National Audit Office in the UK rightly emphasised the priority but it remains to work out how to achieve it in practice.[12]

Cancer as a common disease

Cancer care is often regarded as a province for specialists only: yet with increased numbers of patients and a requirement for longer-term support the role of the primary care team is set to increase. In 2000, a set of guidelines was established for the initial referral of suspected cancer patients, providing detailed guidance on how to identify patients requiring urgent referral. It is now necessary to evaluate whether the guidelines actually achieved the results of earlier detection, although so far, the results for breast cancer look positive. The aspiration is clear enough: what now remains is to carry out more development projects on how to develop it in the most effective way.

We would welcome the opportunity to develop shared-care models, and for cancer centres to involve GPs with special interests. For some types of cancer, such as prostate cancer, some of the initial diagnostic assessment is being carried out in primary care. Clearer protocols and clinical governance standards will make it much easier to involve primary care teams in the cancer journey. Until now, the role of primary care in cancer services has been mainly concerned with palliative care, but there could be a more extensive role in developing care pathways and in monitoring risk.[13]

Increasing choice in treatment

Patient preferences and capabilities are going to become much more important as cancer becomes a longer-term illness with many more elderly patients. The issues of the design and the location of services so as to ensure maximum patient involvement will become a major issue. With more oral chemotherapy it will be possible to develop more local access at community hospitals and primary care centres. For older patients needing radiotherapy it may be possible to redesign programmes or to organise transport to more distant centres. Patients will want to know more about risks and benefits of treatment. Even though anti-emetics have improved the patient experience, there may still be important side-effects from treatment. Some of the symptoms may clear up quite quickly but they will be quite painful. A UK patient has described some experiences:

> On February 3rd 2003, I started 6 weeks of chemo-rad: low dose capecitabine with radiotherapy at 10 a.m. Monday–Friday of each week. This was probably the worst phase of treatment. The capecitabine had to be taken one hour before and 12 hours after each radiotherapy session and I had to ensure that I had a full bladder for the radiotherapy. The first two weeks were fine but after that I suddenly developed proctitis (inflammation of the rectum) with going to the toilet best described as "shitting razor blades!" This was controlled to some extent with steroid cream and local anaesthetic gel but was still very painful. As the six weeks went on I was getting a fair amount of discomfort around the coccyx and found it difficult to walk more than a few hundred yards. At the time, I didn't really realize how tired it was making me: when it finished all the symptoms cleared up in a couple of weeks.

Geographic distribution of treatment centres

Until now, the key issues affecting organisation and location have been those concerned with clinical specialisation and concentration of equipment. These considerations have usually created an irresistible pressure towards concentration of services at a few locations. Of course, such issues remain critical but it is surely time to ensure that evidence can be reviewed on customer/patient perspectives. When patients attend treatment centres many times, convenience of location may start to affect the take-up of therapies quite apart from considerations of patient convenience. Where there is scope for meeting clinical requirements in different ways it is surely time to search for degrees of freedom in how services are designed. In fact, there may be unexpected gains to having more access and treatment at different points. The US system has had multiple access points with treatment much more widely available in physician's offices. Apart from some specialised surgery, there has not been the same pull to specialisation as in the UK where most treatment is being concentrated on as few as 50 hubs. The greater use of web and IT systems such as personal access communication system (PACS), may in fact mean that it would be much more possible to develop networks and to manage treatment programmes on different sites. It will also make it far easier to set consistent standards for quality.

Improving cancer rehabilitation and longer-term support

Cardiac services include a strong element of rehabilitation. The presumption is that most patients can be helped back to the lifestyle of their choice. For the UK, rehabilitation is one key standard in the National Service Framework for Coronary Heart Disease.[14]

As cancer becomes a chronic illness it is surely time to add in rehabilitation as part of the core programme together with advice on future options and financial arrangements. For many patients, cancer is an adverse economic event (even a disaster) as well as a disease. Within the US patients may face heavy costs in funding drug therapies: in Europe economic effects may include loss of employment and inability to get insurance policies or credit. One study in the UK examined the social problems of cancer patients under eight headings.[15] The categories were:

1. problems of managing in the home,
2. health and welfare services,
3. finances,
4. employment,
5. legal matters,
6. relationships,
7. sexuality and body image,
8. recreation.

Most commonly experienced were difficulties in relationships, appearance, and travel or getting around. Women patients experienced somewhat more problems than men, and palliative care patients experienced more than others. It is likely that more such problems will be experienced with longer-term illness and declining general health. Urgent investment in better support is required if cancer is not to be associated with longer-term disability and loss of quality of life.

Palliative care

A review of the international evidence on palliative care in 1999 sets out some of the key aims:

The aim can be a highly positive one – that of securing quality of life and freedom from pain during the last phase. Palliative care holds out the promise of a period before death, which could be lived free from pain, with dignity protected and last opportunities for positive experience. Such an aim is feasible with current drug therapy and the current state of knowledge on pain control.[16]

Yet, so many patients were not getting this support. They often faced pain, anxiety and loss of dignity in the last phase of life. Since then there have been some positive developments. Hospice care has continued to expand albeit in somewhat different forms in the US and UK. The new development has been the rapid expansion of palliative care with community hospitals in the US. There are now strong economic incentives to develop palliative care.

Cost of palliative care at Virginia Commonwealth Medical centre

	Non-PCU* days (cost $)	PCU*days (cost $)
Drugs and chemotherapy	2267	511
Laboratory tests	1134	56
Diagnostic imaging	615	29
Medical supplies	1821	731
Room and nursing	4330	3708
Other	2152	278
Total	**12,319**	**5313**

*PCU stands for palliative care unit. Each figure represents cost of last 5 days for cancer patients aged 65+ prior to in hospital death. Figures are for 2001 and 2002. *Source*: Naik G. (2004) Palliative care eases variety of pain. *Wall Street Journal*.

Palliative care has expanded rapidly in US hospitals. In 2002, there were palliative care programmes in 844 community hospitals – 18% more than in the previous year. Within the US there are differences between patients in hospice use depending on type of coverage. Patients covered by Medicare managed care were much more likely to be referred to hospices than patients with Medicare fee for service.

Medicare benefici-aries enrolled in managed care had consistently higher rates of hospice use and significantly longer hospice stays than those enrolled in fee for service.[17]

In spite of some improvements there is still a long way to go in ensuring access to palliative care. A report from the National Academies of Science estimated that half of the 550,000 cancer patients who die every year in the USA receive inadequate palliative care. It also showed that the National Cancer Institute (NCI) spent less than 1% of its budget on research in palliative care.[17]

There has been some improvement since, but worldwide palliative care remains a neglected area of healthcare.

Action plans for cancer survivorship

The Lance Armstrong Foundation, founded by the only cancer survivor who has won the Tour de France six times, has been very active in developing an action plan for cancer survivors. Along with the Centre for Disease Control, the Foundation has developed a National Action Plan for Cancer survivors in the US.[18]

Among the key directions are the following:
- Develop an infrastructure for a comprehensive database on cancer survivorship.
- Develop and maintain patient navigation systems that can facilitate optimum care for cancer survivors.
- Establish and maintain patient navigation systems that can facilitate optimum care for cancer survivors.
- Establish and disseminate clinical practice guidelines for each stage of cancer survivorship.
- Develop and disseminate public education programmes that empower cancer survivors to make informed decisions.
- Conduct ongoing evaluation of all activities to determine their impacts and outcomes and ensure continuous quality improvement of services.
- Conduct research on preventive interventions to evaluate their impact on cancer survivorship issues.
- Educate policy- and decision-makers about the role and value of providing long-term follow-up care, addressing quality of life issues and legal needs, and ensuring access to clinical trials and ancillary services for cancer survivors.
- Empower survivors with advocacy skills.
- Educate decision-makers about economic and insurance barriers related to health care for cancer survivors.

- Establish and disseminate guidelines that support quality and timely service provision for cancer services.

The Lance Armstrong Foundation has set an agenda that is relevant across all nations and all income levels. The challenge of improving quality of life for cancer survivors is a new and vital element for the first few years of the 21st century. There is also much to learn from the guidelines on psychosocial care developed in Australia. The guidelines report that up to two-thirds of cancer patients suffer long-term emotional distress and set out ways in which patients can be helped with the emotional and personal fall out from cancer.[19] There can be new international partnerships to develop much better long-term support for cancer patients.

REFERENCES

1. CDC (2004) *Cancer Survivorship – United States, 1971–2001*. CDC, Atlanta.
2. President's Cancer Panel Living Beyond Cancer: a European Dialogue. US department of health and Human Services 2004.
3. Antonio Toscano (2002) *47 Lung Cancer Survivor Diagnosed*. Italy.
4. Fenna Postma-Schit (1978) *60 Thyroid Cancer Survivor Diagnosed*. The Netherlands.
5. Dr Andrew Martin (2004) Personal Communication.
6. Karen Kitzmiller (2001) *Stage 1V Breast Cancer Patient and State Legislator, Vermont (deceased) President's Cancer Panel. Voices of a Broken system*. US Department of Health and Human Services, Washington.
7. Sarna L. et al. (2002) Long term survivors of lung cancer. *Journal Clinical Oncology* 20: 2920–2929.
8. Senior K. (2002) Good quality of life found in long-term breast cancer survivors. *Lancet Oncology* 3(2): 66.
9. Jefford M. and Tattersall M.H.N. (2002) Informing and involving cancer patients in their own care. *Lancet Oncology* 3(10): 629–637.
10. Mills M.E. and Sullivan K. (1999) The importance of information giving for patients newly diagnosed with cancer: a review of the literature. *Journal of Clinical Nursing* 8: 631–642.
11. Pleat J.M., Bailey J. and Dunkin C. (2003) Postoperative web advice for UK patients with breast cancer. *Lancet Oncology* 4(9): 527–528.
12. National Audit Office (2004) *Tackling Cancer in England; Saving More Lives*. London.
13. Leese B. et al. (2004) *"Early Days Yet". The Primary Care Lead Clinician (PCCL) Initiative*. University of Leeds.
14. Doh Coronary Heart Disease (2001) National Service Framework. London.

15. Wright E.P. et al. (2002) Social problems in oncology. *British Journal of Cancer* 87: 1099–1104.

16. Bosanquet N. and Salisbury C. (1999) *Providing a Palliative Care Service Towards an Evidence Base*. OUP, UK.

17. McCarthy E.P. et al. (2003) Hospice use among medicare managed care and fee-for-service patients dying with cancer. *Journal of the American Medical Association* 289: 2238–2245.

18. CDC/Lance Armstrong Foundation (2004) *A National Action Plan for Cancer Survivorship*. Advancing Public Health Strategies, Washington.

19. Howe M. (2003) Australian cancer doctors urged to consider psychosocial care. *The Lancet Oncology* 4(10): 590.

Sources consulted

2020 Vision: *Our Future Healthcare Environments*. 2003. The Stationery Office, Norwich.

American Cancer Society (2004) *Cancer Facts and Figures*. Atlanta.

Blackledge G. (2003) Cancer drugs: the next ten years. *European Journal of Cancer* 39: 273.

Bosanquet N. and Sikora K. (2004) Cancer care in Britain: the economic future. *Lancet Oncology* 9: 568–574.

Breast Cancer Care (2003) *Breast Cancer in the UK. What's the Prognosis?* London.

Brumley R.D. (2002) Future of end of life care: the managed care organisation perspective. *Journal of Palliative Medicine* 5: 263–270.

Butler R. (1997) Population aging and health. *British Medical Journal* 315: 1082–1084.

Cross S.S., Dennis T. and Start R.D. (2002) Telepathology: current status and future prospects in diagnostic histopathology. *Histopathology* 41: 91–109.

Cutler D. and McClellan M. (2001) Is technological change worth it? *Health Affairs* 20: 11–29.

Dargie C. (1999) Demography: analysing trends and policy issues in births, deaths and disease in the UK population in 2015. In: *Policy Futures for UK Health* (ed. Dargie C.). The Nuffield Trust, London.

Dargie C., Dawson S. and Garside P. (2000) *Policy Futures for UK Health*: 2000 Report. The Nuffield Trust, London.

Department of Health (1995) *Recommendations for Commissioning Cancer Services; Report of the Expert Advisory Group on Cancer*. London.

Department of Health (2000) *Shaping the Future NHS: Long Term Planning for Hospitals and Related Services*. Department of Health, London.

Dixon J., Le Grand J. and Smith P. (2003) *Shaping the New NHS: Can Market Forces be Used for Good?* King's Fund, London.

Herzlinger R. (1997) *Market Driven Health Care*. Addison Wesley, Massachusetts.

Holtzman N.A. and Shapiro D. (1998) Genetic testing and public policy. *British Medical Journal* 316: 852–856.

ICRF (1995) *Our Vision for Cancer*. ICRF, London.

Imperial Cancer Research Fund (1995) *A Vision for Cancer*. Imperial Cancer Research Fund, London.

Institute of Medicine (2001) Crossing the Quality Chasm: A New Health System for the 21st Century. National Academy Press, Washington, USA.

Introcaso D. and Lynn J. (2002) Systems of care: future reform. *Journal of Palliative Medicine* 5: 255–257.

Kendall L. (2001) *The Future Patient.* IPPR, London.

Kirkwood T. (2003) The most pressing problem of our age. *British Medical Journal* 326: 1297–1299.

Laing A. (2002) Meeting patient expectations: healthcare professionals and service re-engineering. *Health Services Management Research* 15: 165–172.

Lissauer R. and Kendall L. (2002) New practitioners in the future health service: exploring roles for practitioners in primary and intermediate care. IPPR, London.

Locock L. (2003) Healthcare redesign: meanings, origins and application. *Quality and Safety in Health Care* 12: 53–58.

Locock L. (2003) Redesigning health care: new wine from old bottles? *Journal of Health Services Research and Policy* 8: 120–122.

Melzer D. (2003) *My Very Own Medicine: What Must I Know?* Department of Public Health, University of Cambridge, Cambridge.

Morris K. (2003) 10 years and counting: the hype and hope of cancer biotechnology. *The Lancet* 3: 582.

Murray C.J. and Lopez A.D. (1996) Baseline projections of HIV incidence and mortality by region. In: *The Global Burden of Disease.* Harvard University Press, Boston, pp. 348–352.

Murray C.J. and Lopez A.D. (1996) The global burden of disease. Harvard University Press, Boston.

Nicolette C.A. and Miller G.A. (2003) The identification of clinically relevant markers and therapeutic targets. *Drug Discovery Today* 8: 31–38.

OECD (2003) *Health Care Systems: Lessons from the Reform Experience.* OECD, Paris.

Parish C. (2002) Tomorrow's cancer. *Nursing Standard* 17(1): 12–13.

Peckham M. and Lee M. (2001) *Health Trends Review.* Department of Health, London.

Richards C., Dinwall R. and Watson A. (2001) Should NHS patients be allowed to contribute extra money to their care? *British Medical Journal* 323: 563–565.

Sikora K. (1999) Developing a global strategy for cancer. *European Journal of Cancer* 11: 368–370.

Sikora K. (2000) The future of cancer care. *The Pharmacia Lecture.* Pharmacia Publications, New York.

Sikora K. (2002) The impact of future technology on cancer care. *Clinical Medicine* 2: 560–568.

Sikora K. and Bosanquet N. (2003) Cancer care in the United Kingdom: new solutions are needed. *British Medical Journal* 327: 1044–1046.

Singh G., O'Donoghue J. and Kee Soon C. (2002) Telemedicine: issues and implications. *Technology and Health Care* 10: 1–10.

Social Market Foundation Health Commission (2002) *User Charges: Shifting the Costs to Consumers*. London.

Symonds R. P. (2001) Radiotherapy. *British Medical Journal* 323: 1107–1110.

Tritter J.Q. and Calnan N. (2002) Cancer as a chronic illness? Reconsidering categorisation and exploring experience. *European Journal of Cancer* 11: 161–165.

Wanless D. (2002) Securing our future health: taking the long-term view. Department of Health, London.

Wanless D. (2003) Securing good health for the whole population. Department of Health, London.

Watters J.W. and McLeod H.L. (2003) Cancer pharmacogenomics: current and future applications. *Biochimica et Biophysica Acta* 1603: 99–111.

West E. (2003) *Nursing Workforce Issues*. Macmillan Cancer Relief, London.

WHO (1998) *The World Health Report*. WHO, Geneva.

WHO (2003) *World Cancer Report*. IARC, Lyons.

WHO-IARC (1998) *Electronic Database for Cancer in 5 Continents*. WHO-IARC, Lyon.

World Cancer Report (2003) IARC Press, Lyons.

Yabroff R. et al. (2004) Burden of illness in cancer survivors; findings from a population-based national sample. *Journal of National Cancer Institute* 96: 1322–1330.

Index

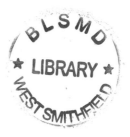